Laboratory Procedures in Clinical Veterinary Bacteriology

G. W. Osbaldiston, Ph.D., B.V.Sc.
Yale University School of Medicine

University Park Press
Baltimore · London · Tokyo

UNIVERSITY PARK PRESS
International Publishers in Science and Medicine
Chamber of Commerce Building
Baltimore, Maryland 21202

Printed in the United States of America

Library of Congress Cataloging in Publication Data

Osbaldiston, G.W.
Laboratory procedures in clinical veterinary bacteriology.

1. Veterinary bacteriology—Technique. I. Title.
QR49.078 636.089'69'2 72-13530
ISBN 0-8391-0610-6

Laboratory Procedures in Clinical Veterinary Bacteriology

Preface

This volume provides a system of clinical bacteriology which is simple, reliable, and practical for the veterinarian's office, but sufficiently sophisticated to establish the identity of potential pathogens of domestic animals.

The system has been evolved over a period of years in my laboratory. It is comprised of two parts. The first part requires only simple media and few reagents, which give clearcut results with common bacteria. These basic procedures are outlined in Figure 2, pp. 32–34. From the results of these simple tests, a bacterial isolate can be placed into a small group of genera, from which tentative identification can be made if the host animal and the site of isolation are known. For clinical purposes, this degree of identification is usually sufficient.

For precise identification, a series of more elaborate tests are given. This comprises the second part of the system.

The old saying, "When you hear hoofbeats don't think of zebras," is pertinent in bacteriology. In a series of 3,000 bacterial cultures from domestic animals, in my laboratory, the following 11 genera constituted approximately 85% of the isolations: *Escherichia, Enterobacter, Salmonella, Pasteurella, Klebsiella, Pseudomonas, Proteus, Streptococcus, Staphylococcus, Corynebacterium,* and *Clostridium.* The beginner would be well advised to develop confidence in techniques for isolating these genera first.

There are two excellent textbooks on veterinary bacteriology, *Veterinary Bacteriology and Virology,* by Drs. I. A. Merchant and R. A. Packer of the College of Veterinary Medicine, Iowa State University, and *Infectious Diseases of Domestic Animals,* by Drs. D. W. Brunner and J. H. Gillespie of the New York State Veterinary College, Cornell

University. These texts are recommended to all readers. It is my hope that this volume will supply the practical dimension to complement these other books.

It is a pleasure to acknowledge the assistance of Mr. E. C. Stowe and Mrs. W. S. Walker, whose help in formulating the ideas presented in the volume and in testing their practical application has been invaluable.

G. W. O.

Contents

1

Introduction

Clinical bacteriology is that aspect of microbiology that deals with the recognition of pathogenic bacteria and their differentiation from the normal flora. Most bacteriology textbooks are systematically organized around some general property of each organism. This book is organized around the practical aspects of the isolation and recognition of potentially pathogenic bacteria from the usual specimens obtained in veterinary medicine.

1. Importance of Clinical Bacteriology in Veterinary Medicine

The results of bacterial examination are used in confirming diagnosis, establishing prognosis, and selecting effective treatment.

Most individual sick animals are seen on an outpatient basis. Bacterial infection in such patients usually responds well to the appropriate antibiotic therapy, because marked drug resistance is comparatively rare. Cases of otitis externa, cystitis, and pyoderma, however, are notoriously difficult to treat, and successful therapy depends on identification of the bacteria involved and establishment of in vitro antibiotic susceptibility. With animals hospitalized because of severe illness or surgical problems, complete bacteriological examination is necessary. These animals do not readily respond to therapy because their specific defense mechanisms against infection are depressed as a result of excessive endogenous steroid secretion or the administration of large doses of synthetic steroids. This applies, for instance, to horses infected with Salmonellosis, which is often a sequel to major surgery.

The importance of bacteriology in medical problems affecting groups of animals cannot be overstressed. For example, bacterial identification and antibiotic sensitivity studies are an integral part of a mastitis control program. The economics of the treatment of infectious diseases in intensively cared-for animals justifies bacterial examination, since incorrect therapy or inadequate disease control measures caused by inaccurate diagnosis can have serious financial consequences.

Bacterial investigation should be performed on any species in the following situations: (a) acute illness or febrile reaction, (b) sudden death, (c) infection or abortion, (d) diarrhea, and (e) inflammatory reactions with exudate formation.

Bacteriology is fundamental in the areas of epidemiology and veterinary public health. Correct identification of all organisms involved in a problem is essential. This rapidly expanding area of veterinary medicine requires the active participation of all veterinarians with access to bacteriological facilities.

2. The Practical Problem

At present very few veterinary practices have their own bacteriology laboratories. This is not attributable to lack of interest by the veterinary profession or to the absence of the need for bacteriological examinations; it occurs simply because in the teaching of bacteriology the practical aspects of the isolation and identification of organisms from clinical specimens has not been emphasized.

When bacterial disease is suspected in an animal, the common procedure is to collect a specimen, initiate therapy, and then send the specimen to a laboratory. Often the clinician concerns himself with the antibiotic sensitivity result, since the decision to continue or to change therapy is based on this information. This result is important in an outpatient clinic, since it takes from several days to a week for bacterial identification to be completed. While it is clinically expedient to be concerned solely with antibiotic susceptibility, in most cases it is poor medical practice. Without identification of the agent, antibiotic sensitivity results may be clinically invalid. They may, for example, relate to an organism other than the one responsible for the infection.

In order to proceed most effectively with the treatment of an infectious disease, the veterinary clinician must know whether bacterial infection is involved and, if so, the identification and chemotherapeutic sensitivity of the organism. The primary function of the clinical bacteriology laboratory is, therefore, to provide presumptive bacterial identification and antibiograms quickly and accurately. For clinical purposes, identification of the genus of the bacteria is sufficient for the initiation of treatment and the establishment of prognosis.

3. Objectives

The objective of this work is to describe a system of veterinary clinical bacteriology in sufficient detail to enable any veterinarian to develop an adequate laboratory. The system is designed for two levels of operation: first, for the practitioner's use in his office, and, second, for use in the diagnostic laboratory for final identification of organisms.

4. Outline of the System

As the first step in this system, the specimen to be identified is lightly streaked onto blood agar and MacConkey agar. After incubation at 37°C for 24 hr, the culture plates are examined for colony growth. Individual colonies representing each colony type growing on the plate are inoculated into tubes of triple sugar iron (TSI) agar and incubated overnight. From the reaction of TSI agar, growth on the initial medium, gram stain and catalase reactions, presumptive identification of the isolates can be made. With anaerobic organisms it is best to allow from 48 to 72 hr for initial culturing time. Once an organism is obtained in pure culture, its identity can be established by testing for specific reactions.

5. Procedures for Collecting Specimens

The initial step in identification of bacterial isolates is to culture the specimen on blood and MacConkey agar plates. Therefore, when an animal is examined, sterile culture plates containing these agars, sterile cotton swabs, and a marking pencil (chinagraph) should be on hand.

The steps involved in culturing a specimen are as follows:

1. At the start of each day a number of blood and MacConkey agar culture plates are removed from refrigerated storage. The plates of each type are stacked one on top of another. For ease of handling, a strip of masking tape is attached to each side of the stack. The plates will not become contaminated if kept this way, and can conveniently be

transported in an equipment bag or left in an examination room. When a culture plate is needed, the tape on one side of the stack is loosened, the plate lifted off, inoculated, and then returned to the stack and secured with the tape.

2. The specimen is collected on a sterile cotton swab and immediately placed on one plate of each type. Experience has shown that it is more satisfactory to take the plates to the animal than to collect the specimen and transport it in a sterile vial to the laboratory for plating at a later time. In farm animal medicine, sterile culture plates can be carried easily and safely in an equipment bag. The direct plating of a specimen can conveniently be done in a stall or field with no more risk of contamination than there is when plating the specimen in a sterile vial. As soon as a culture plate has been used, it is identified by marking the bottom with a chinagraph pencil. The plate is then returned to the stack and secured.

3. The inoculated plates are then ready for incubation. The plates may be held for up to 48 hr before incubation, provided the lids are firmly held down. In farm animal practice the plates are incubated at 37°C on return to the hospital. In companion animal practice the plates are transferred to the incubator at any convenient time.

4. At the end of the day unused sterile plates are returned to the refrigerator for storage.

6. Presumptive Identification of Bacteria

For presumptive identification of bacteria, the following information is required: (1) ability to grow on blood and/or MacConkey agar, (2) color of colonies on MacConkey agar, (3) glucose utilization or H_2S production in TSI agar, (4) catalase reaction, (5) gram stain, (6) site of isolation, and (7) host animal. In Chapter 5, Figure 1 (page 30) bacteria are grouped according to criteria 1 through 5 above. When the tests on an unknown organism have been completed, apply the results to Figure 1 and place the organism in its correct group. For presumptive identification of the organism, the information in Section 2 is required also. Here the bacteria are numbered, and the numbers in Figure 2 (pages 32–34) correspond with those in Section 2 of Chapter 5. Check each organism from the specific group in Figure 2 with respect to site of isolation and host species with the information in Section 2.

The steps for presumptive recognition of bacteria are simple to perform and give clear-cut results. Thus nonprofessional office staff can quickly learn how to perform a bacterial identification. This is an important advantage to the veterinarian who does not have the work load to support a laboratory technologist. Identification can be made within 48 hr of collection of the specimen, and with a little experience many shortcuts can be introduced so that identification can often be made within one day after inoculation.

7. Definitive Identification of Bacteria

Section 2 of Chapter 5 contains typical biochemical reactions that can be used to differentiate organisms within a group. With such specific information, precise identification can be made.

Exact identification should not be expected in all instances. Some bacteria, especially the gram-negative enteric bacteria, occasionally have atypical reactions. In Section 2 reactions showing the minimum variation have been selected, but it would be naive to suggest that the scheme is absolute. The procedures in use in the author's laboratory form the basis for this presentation, and experience has shown that only rarely can precise identification not be made.

2

Bacterial Diseases of Domestic Animals

In listing the bacterial diseases of animals, the author's intention has been to provide a source of reference for the potential isolates from various sites.

1. Bacterial Diseases of Cats

Site	Disease	Organism	Gram reaction	Morphology
Blood	septicemia	*Clostridium chauvoei*	+	bacillus
		Streptococcus pyogenes	+	coccus
Lung	hemorrhagic septicemia	*Pasteurella multocida*	–	bacillus
	melioidosis	*Pseudomonas pseudomallei*	–	bacillus
	nocardiosis	*Nocardia asteroides*	+	branching filaments
	pneumonia	*Hemophilus influenzae*	–	bacillus
		Bordetella bronchiseptica	–	bacillus
		Streptococcus pyogenes	+	coccus
Throat	anthrax	*Bacillus anthracis*	+	bacillus
Intestine and feces	enteritis	*Escherichia coli*	–	bacillus
		Salmonella anatum	–	bacillus
		Salmonella cholerae-suis	–	bacillus
		Salmonella typhimurium	–	bacillus
Mammary glands	enterotoxemia	*Clostridium perfringens*	+	bacillus
	mastitis	*Escherichia coli*	–	bacillus

Site	Disease	Organism	Gram reaction	Morphology
Mammary glands—*Cont'd*		*Staphylococcus aureus*	+	coccus
		Streptococcus pyogenes	+	coccus
Urine	cystitis	*Escherichia coli*	–	bacillus
		Proteus mirabilis	–	bacillus
		Peptococcus sp.	+	coccus
		Staphylococcus aureus	+	coccus
		Peptostreptococcus sp.	+	coccus
		Streptococcus pyogenes	+	coccus
		Corynebacterium acnes	+	bacillus
Skin	botryomycosis	*Micrococcus ascoformans*	+	coccus
	lockjaw	*Clostridium tetani*	+	bacillus
	wounds	*Proteus mirabilis*	–	bacillus
		Pasteurella multocida	–	bacillus
		Pseudomonas aeruginosa	–	bacillus
		Staphylococcus aureus	+	coccus
		Streptococcus pyogenes	+	coccus
		Actinomyces baudeti	+	bacillus
Eyes	conjunctivitis	*Moraxella* spp.	–	coccus
Blood and parenchymatous organs, kittens	neonatal mortality	*Escherichia coli*	–	bacillus
		Salmonella anatum	–	bacillus
		Salmonella typhimurium	–	bacillus
		Streptococcus pyogenes	+	coccus

2. Bacterial Diseases of Dogs

Blood	anthrax	*Bacillus anthracis*	+	bacillus
	hemorrhagic septicemia	*Pasteurella multocida*	–	bacillus
	septicemia	*Pasteurella haemolytica*	–	bacillus
Lung	hemorrhagic septicemia	*Pasteurella multocida*	–	bacillus
	septicemia	*Pasteurella haemolytica*	–	bacillus
	meliodosis	*Pseudomonas pseudomallei*	–	bacillus
	nocardiosis	*Nocardia asteroides*	+	branching filaments
	pneumonia	*Bordetella bronchiseptica*	–	bacillus
		Klebsiella pneumoniae	–	bacillus
		Pseudomonas aeruginosa	–	bacillus
		Staphylococcus aureus	+	coccus

Site	Disease	Organism	Gram reaction	Morphology
Lung—*Cont'd*		*Streptococcus pyogenes*	+	coccus
		Pasteurella tularensis	–	bacillus
	tuberculosis	*Mycobacterium tuberculosis*	+	bacillus
		Mycobacterium bovis	+	bacillus
Intestine	enteritis	*Salmonella bredeney*	–	bacillus
		Salmonella newport	–	bacillus
		Salmonella typhimurium	–	bacillus
		Salmonella dublin	–	bacillus
		Enterococcus	–	coccus
		Staphylococcus sp.	+	coccus
		Escherichia coli	–	bacillus
		Proteus mirabilis	–	bacillus
Fetus and genital tract	abortion	*Brucella canis*	–	bacillus
		Clostridium septicum	+	bacillus
	metritis	*Brucella abortus*	–	bacillus
		Escherichia coli	–	bacillus
		Staphylococcus aureus	+	coccus
	pyometra	*Streptococcus pyogenes*	+	coccus
		Staphylococcus aureus	+	coccus
		Escherichia coli	–	bacillus
Mammary glands	mastitis	*Staphylococcus aureus*	+	coccus
		Proteus mirabilis	–	bacillus
		Enterobacter aerogenes	–	bacillus
Urine	cystitis	*Peptococcus* sp.	+	coccus
		Peptostreptococcus sp.	+	coccus
		Escherichia coli	–	bacillus
		Pseudomonas aeruginosa	–	bacillus
		Proteus mirabilis	–	bacillus
		Corynebacterium renale	+	bacillus
		Streptococcus pyogenes	–	coccus
	leptospirosis	*Leptospira canicola*	Giemsa	spirillum
		Leptospira icterohaemorrhagica	Giemsa	spirillum
Skin	abscess	*Norcardia asteroides*	+	branching filaments
	lockjaw	*Clostridium tetani*	+	bacillus
	pyoderma	*Corynebacterium* spp. (anaerobic)	+	bacillus
		Staphylococcus aureus	+	coccus
		Streptococcus pyogenes	+	coccus
Ears	otitis externa	*Streptococcus pyogenes*	+	coccus

Site	Disease	Organism	Gram reaction	Morphology
Ears—*Cont'd*		*Staphylococcus aureus*	+	coccus
		Pseudomonas aeruginosa	−	bacillus
		Proteus mirabilis	−	bacillus
		Escherichia coli	−	bacillus
Mouth	trench mouth	*Fusobacterium fusiforme*	−	bacillus
		Borrelia vincentii	−	spirillum
Tonsil	tonsilitis	*Streptococcus pyogenes*	+	coccus
Cerebrospinal fluid, brain	encephalitis	*Listeria monocytogenes*	+	bacillus
Eyes	conjunctivitis	*Staphylococcus aureus*	+	coccus
		Pseudomonas aeruginosa	−	bacillus
Blood and parenchymatous organs, puppies	neonatal mortality	*Escherichia coli*	−	bacillus
		Staphylococcus aureus	+	coccus
		Streptococcus pyogenes	+	coccus
		Pseudomonas aeruginosa	−	bacillus

3. Bacterial Diseases of Horses

Blood	anthrax	*Bacillus anthracis*	+	bacillus
	fever	*Coxiella burneti*	−	pleomorphic bacillus
	septicemia	*Actinobacillus equuli*	−	bacillus
Lung	glanders	*Actinobacillus mallei*	−	bacillus
	meloidosis	*Pseudomonas pseudomallei*	−	bacillus
	influenzal pneumonia	*Bordetella bronchiseptica*	−	bacillus
		Streptococcus pyogenes	+	coccus
		Corynebacterium equi	+	bacillus
		Pasteurella multocida	−	bacillus
	tuberculosis	*Mycobacterium tuberculosis*	+	bacillus
Intestine	botulism	*Clostridium botulinum*	+	bacillus
	enteritis	*Escherichia coli*	−	bacillus
		Salmonella typhimurium	−	bacillus
		Salmonella anatum	−	bacillus
	meloidosis	*Pseudomonas pseudomallei*	−	bacillus
	ulceration of intestine	*Sphaerophorus necrophorus*	−	pleomorphic bacillus

Site	Disease	Organism	Gram reaction	Morphology
Fetus and uterus	abortion	*Escherichia coli*	–	bacillus
		Klebsiella pneumoniae var. *genitalium*	–	bacillus
		Actinobacillus equuli	–	bacillus
		Corynebacterium equi	+	bacillus
Mammary glands	mastitis	*Escherichia coli*	–	bacillus
		Staphylococcus aureus	+	coccus
		Streptococcus equi	+	coccus
		Streptococcus zooepidemicus	+	coccus
Urine	cystitis	*Leptospira pomona*	Giemsa	spirillum
		Leptospira hyos	Giemsa	spirillum
		Escherichia coli	–	bacillus
	purulent nephritis	*Actinobacillus equuli*	–	bacillus
	pyelonephritis	*Corynebacterium renale*	+	bacillus
Skin and muscle	fistulous withers	*Brucella abortus*	–	bacillus
	poll evil	*Actinomyces bovis*	+	branching filaments
	lockjaw	*Clostridium tetani*	+	bacillus
	malignant edema	*Clostridium septicum*	+	bacillus
	necrotic dermatitis	*Sphaerophorus necrophorus*	–	pleomorphic bacillus
	strangles	*Streptococcus equi*	+	coccus
	ulcerative lymphangitis	*Corynebacterium pseudotuberculosis*	+	bacillus
	wounds	*Streptococcus pyogenes*	+	coccus
		Peptostreptococcus spp.	+	bacillus
		Bacteroides spp.	+	bacillus
		Proteus mirabilis	–	bacillus
		Pseudomonas aeruginosa	–	bacillus
		Actinobacillus mallei	–	bacillus
Joint	joint ill	*Actinobacillus equuli*	–	bacillus
		Corynebacterium equi	+	bacillus
		Escherichia coli	–	bacillus

Site	Disease	Organism	Gram reaction	Morphology
Blood and parenchymatous organs, foals	neonatal mortality	*Streptococcus zooepidemicus*	+	coccus
		Streptococcus equisimilis	+	coccus
		Streptococcus equi	+	coccus
		Actinobacillus equuli	−	bacillus
		Salmonella abortus-equi	−	bacillus
		Escherichia coli	−	bacillus
		Klebsiella pneumoniae var. *genitalium*	−	bacillus

4. Bacterial Diseases of Cattle

Blood	anthrax	*Bacillus anthracis*	−	bacillus
	shipping fever	*Pasteurella multocida*	−	bacillus
		Pasteurella haemolytica	−	bacillus
		Yersinia pseudotuberculosis	−	bacillus
Lung	calf necrotic diphtheria	*Sphaerophorus necrophorus*	−	pleomorphic bacillus
	contagious bovine pleuropneumonia	*Mycoplasma mycoides*	Giemsa	pleomorphic forms
	nocardiosis	*Nocardia asteroides*	+	branching filaments
	pneumonia	*Hemophilus bovis*	−	bacillus
		Diplococcus pneumoniae	+	diplococcus
	shipping fever	*Pasteurella multocida*	−	bacillus
		Pasteurella hemolytica	−	bacillus
	tuberculosis	*Mycobacterium tuberculosis*	+	bacillus
Liver	infectious necrosis hepatitis	*Clostridium novyi*	+	bacillus
	necrotic abscesses	*Sphaerophorus necrophorus*	−	pleomorphic bacillus
	redwater	*Clostridium hemolyticum*	+	bacillus
	septicemia	*Achromobacter anitratum*	−	coccobacillus
Intestine	calf scours	*Clostridium perfringens* Type C	+	bacillus
		Escherichia coli	−	bacillus

Site	Disease	Organism	Gram reaction	Morphology
Intestine—*Cont'd*	enteritis	*Salmonella typhimurium*	–	bacillus
		Salmonella dublin	–	bacillus
		Salmonella newport	–	bacillus
		Salmonella anatum	–	bacillus
		Salmonella arizona	–	bacillus
	hemorrhagic enterotoxemia	*Clostridium perfringens* Type C	+	bacillus
	Johne's disease	*Mycobacterium paratuberculosis*	+	bacillus
	necrosis of rumen	*Sphaerophorus necrophorus*	–	pleomorphic bacillus
Fetus and uterus	abortion	*Brucella abortus*	–	bacillus
		Vibrio fetus	–	curved
		Corynebacterium pyogenes	+	bacillus
		Listeria monocytogenes	+	bacillus
Udder	mastitis	*Staphylococcus aureus*	+	coccus
		Streptococcus agalactiae	+	coccus
		Streptococcus uberus	+	coccus
		Streptococcus dysgalactiae	+	coccus
		Streptococcus pyogenes	+	coccus
		Diplococcus pneumoniae	+	coccus
		Escherichia coli	–	bacillus
		Proteus mirabilis	–	bacillus
		Enterobacter aerogenes	–	bacillus
		Pseudomonas aeruginosa	–	bacillus
		Alcaligenes faecalis	–	bacillus
		Corynebacterium pyogenes	+	bacillus
		Klebsiella pneumoniae	–	bacillus
		Sphaerophorus necrophorus	–	pleomorphic bacillus
Urine	cystitis	*Escherichia coli*	–	bacillus
	leptospirosis	*Leptospira pomona*	Giemsa	spirillum
		Leptospira sejroc phosa	Giemsa	spirillum
		Leptospira hyos	Giemsa	spirillum
		Leptospira icterohaemorrhagiae	Giemsa	spirillum
		Leptospira canicola	Giemsa	spirillum
	nephritis	*Sphaerophorus necrophorus*		pleomorphic bacillus
	pyelonephritis	*Corynebacterium renale*	+	bacillus

Site	Disease	Organism	Gram reaction	Morphology
Skin and muscle	big head, wooden tongue	*Actinobacillus lignieresi*	−	bacillus
	blackleg	*Clostridium chauvoei*	+	bacillus
	foot rot	*Sphaerophorus necrophorus*	−	pleomorphic bacillus
	lumpy jaw	*Actinomyces bovis*	+	pleomorphic filaments
	malignant edema	*Clostridium septicum*	+	bacillus
	pyobacillosis	*Corynebacterium pyogenes*	+	coccobacillus
Joints	arthritis	*Erysipelothrix insidiosa*	+	bacillus
Eyes	infectious keratitis	*Moraxella bovis*	−	coccobacillus
Cerebrospinal fluid, brain	listeriosis	*Listeria monocytogenes*	+	bacillus
	encephalitis	*Achromobacter anitratum*	−	coccobacillus
Blood and parenchymatous organs, calves	neonatal mortality	*Escherichia coli*	−	bacillus
		Streptococcus pyogenes	+	coccus
		Pasteurella multocida	−	bacillus
		Cornynebacterium pyogenes	+	bacillus
		Clostridium perfringens	+	bacillus

5. Bacterial Diseases of Sheep

Blood	anthrax	*Bacillus anthracis*	+	bacillus
	Black's disease	*Clostridium novyi*	+	
		Salmonella typhimurium	−	bacillus
	septicemia	*Pasteurella multocida*	−	bacillus
	shipping fever	*Pasteurella hemolytica*	−	bacillus
	tularemia	*Pasteurella tularensis*	−	bacillus
Liver	necrotic hepatitis	*Sphaerophorus necrophorus*	−	bacillus

Site	Disease	Organism	Gram reaction	Morphology
Liver—*Cont'd*	septicemia	*Achromobacter anitratum*	–	cocco-bacillus
Lungs	meliodosis	*Pseudomonas pseudomallei*	–	bacillus
	pneumonia	*Pasteurella hemolytica*	–	bacillus
		Corynebacterium pyogenes	+	bacillus
		Corynebacterium equi	+	bacillus
		Mycobacterium bovis	+	bacillus
Intestine	Botulism	*Clostridium botulinum*	+	bacillus
	enteritis	*Salmonella typhimurium*	–	bacillus
	enterotoxemia, pulpy kidney	*Clostridium perfringens*	+	bacillus
	Johne's disease	*Mycobacterium paratuberculosis*	+	bacillus
	lamb dysentry	*Clostridium perfringens*	+	bacillus
	vibriosis	*Vibrio jejuni*	–	curved bacillus
Fetus and genital tract	abortion	*Brucella ovis*	–	bacillus
		Brucella melitensis	–	bacillus
		Vibrio fetus	–	curved bacillus
		Corynebacterium pseudotuberculosis	+	bacillus
		Streptococcus fecalis	+	coccus
		Salmonella arizonae	–	bacillus
		Salmonella typhimurium	–	bacillus
		Pasteurella hemolytica	–	bacillus
Udder	mastitis	*Staphylococcus aureus*	+	coccus
		Streptococcus zooepidemicus	+	coccus
		Pasteurella hemolytica	–	bacillus
		Corynebacterium pyogenes	+	bacillus
		Enterococcus	–	coccus
		Enterobacter aerogenes	–	bacillus
		Klebsiella pneumoniae var. *genitalium*	–	bacillus
		Brucella abortus	–	bacillus
		Mycoplasma agalactiae	Giemsa	pleomorphic
Urine	cystitis	*Proteus mirabilis*	–	bacillus
		Pseudomonas aeruginosa	–	bacillus

Site	Disease	Organism	Gram reaction	Morphology
Urine—*Cont'd*	pyelonephritis	*Corynebacterium renale*	+	bacillus
Skin and muscle	abscess	*Proteus mirabilis*	–	bacillus
		Staphylococcus aureus	+	coccus
		Pseudomonas aeroginosa	–	bacillus
		Sphaerophorus necrophorus	–	pleomorphic bacillus
	actinobacillosis	*Actinobacillus lignieresi*	–	bacillus
	blackleg	*Clostridium chauvoei*	+	bacillus
	cheesy gland	*Corynebacterium ovis*	+	bacillus
	foot rot	*Sphaerophorus nodosus*	–	pleomorphic bacillus
	lockjaw	*Clostridium tetani*	+	bacillus
	malignant edema	*Clostridium septicum*	+	bacillus
	pyobacillosis	*Corynebacterium pyogenes*	+	bacillus
	swelled head	*Clostridium novyi*	+	bacillus
Eye	pink eye	*Colesiota conjunctivae*	Giemsa	bacillus
Cerebrospinal fluid	listeriosis	*Listeria monocytogenes*	+	bacillus
Blood and parenchymatous organs, lambs	neonatal mortality	*Escherichia coli*	–	bacillus
		Spherophorus necrophorus	–	pleomorphic bacillus
		Erysipelothrix insidiosa	+	bacillus
		Corynebacterium pyogenes	+	bacillus
		Staphylococcus aureus	+	coccus
		Clostridium septicum	+	bacillus
		Clostridium chauvoei	+	bacillus
		Clostridium novyi	+	bacillus
		Clostridium perfringens	+	bacillus
		Pasteurella hemolytica	–	bacillus

6. Bacterial Diseases of Pigs

Blood	anthrax	*Bacillus anthracis*	+	bacillus
	endocarditis	*Streptococcus pyogenes*	+	coccus

Site	Disease	Organism	Gram reaction	Morphology
Blood—*Cont'd*	erysipelas	*Erysipelothrix insidiosa*	+	bacillus
	hemorrhagic septicemia	*Pasteurella multocida*	–	bacillus
		Pasteurella hemolytica	–	bacillus
	meloidosis	*Pseudomonas pseudomallei*	–	bacillus
	septicemia	*Achrombacter anitratium*	–	cocco-bacillus
Liver	enzootic pneumonia	*Mycoplasma hyopneumoniae*	Giemsa	pleomorphic forms
Lung	pneumonia	*Pasteurella multocida*	–	bacillus
		Bordetella bronchiseptica	–	bacillus
		Haemophilus suis	–	bacillus
	botulism	*Clostridium botulinum*	+	bacillus
	dysentery	*Vibrio coli*	–	curved bacillus
Intestine	enteritis	*Salmonella typhimurium*	–	bacillus
		Salmonella cholerae-suis	–	bacillus
		Salmonella anatum	–	bacillus
	edema disease	*Escherichia coli*	–	bacillus
	ulcers	*Sphaerophorus necrophorus*	–	pleomorphic bacillus
Fetus and genital tract	abortion	*Brucella suis*	–	bacillus
		Brucella abortus	–	bacillus
		Salmonella typhimurium	–	bacillus
		Listeria monocytogenes	+	bacillus
Mammary gland	mastitis	*Staphylococcus aureus*	+	coccus
		Streptococcus agalactiae	+	coccus
		Streptococcus uberis	+	coccus
		Escherichia coli	–	bacillus
		Klebsiella pneumoniae	–	bacillus
		Corynebacterium pyogenes	+	bacillus
		Sphaerophorus necrophorus	–	pleomorphic bacillus
	udder abscess	*Actinobacillus lignieresi*	–	bacillus
Urine	cystitis	*Escherichia coli*	–	bacillus
		Staphylococcus aureus	+	coccus
	leptospirosis	*Leptospira pomona*	Giemsa	spirillum

Site	Disease	Organism	Gram reaction	Morphology
Urine—*Cont'd*		*Leptospira hyos*	Giemsa	spirillum
		Leptospira grippotyphosa	Giemsa	spirillum
		Leptospira autumnalis	Giemsa	spirillum
Skin and muscles	abscess	*Streptococcus zooepidemicus*	+	coccus
		Streptococcus equisimilis	+	coccus
		Sphaerophorus necrophorus	–	pleomorphic bacillus
	lockjaw	*Clostridium tetani*	+	bacillus
	lumpy jaw	*Actinomyces bovis*	–	branching filaments
	malignant edema	*Clostridium septicum*	+	bacillus
	wooden tongue	*Actinobacillus lignieresi*	–	bacillus
	wounds	*Proteus mirabilis*	–	bacillus
		Staphylococcus aureus	+	coccus
		Corynebacterium pyogenes	+	bacillus
		Pasteurella multocida	–	bacillus
		Sphaerophorus necrophorus	–	pleomorphic bacillus
Joints	arthritis	*Mycoplasma hyorhinis*	Giemsa	pleomorphic forms
Blood and parenchymatous organs, piglets	neonatal mortality	*Escherichia coli*	–	bacillus
		Erysipelothrix insidiosa	+	bacillus
		Streptococcus zooepidemicus	+	coccus
		Brucella suis	–	bacillus

3

Collection and Handling of Specimens

The collection of the specimen is the most important step of the entire procedure for identification of bacteria. (This point, regretably, is not often appreciated by clinicians, who frequently delegate this responsibility to junior students.) Transfer of the specimen to the culture medium immediately after collection is the best procedure. Transfer into sterile vials for transport to the laboratory (for subsequent plating) should be avoided whenever possible. If a few simple precautions are taken, culture plates should not become contaminated when taken to the animal for immediate plating. With organisms requiring anaerobic conditions, culture plates should be placed in this environment as soon as possible after inoculation. If this cannot be done within a few hours, the specimen should be inoculated into thioglycolate broth.

The preferred methods for the collection and handling of specimens for bacteriological investigation are as follows.

1. *Blood culture*. Clip the hair over the site of venipuncture and clean the skin thoroughly with soap or detergent. Wipe the skin with cotton soaked in alcohol or, preferably, in a solution of 90% alcohol and 10% acetone. In small animals collect 1–2 ml of blood using an aseptic technique and inoculate the specimen into 8–10 ml of thioglycolate broth. Whenever possible, collect 10 ml of blood and inoculate it into 90 ml of medium, since there may be few organisms. Incubate for 24–48 hr and then subculture onto blood and MacConkey agar plates.

2. *Cerebrospinal fluid culture*. Collect at least 1 ml of fluid and proceed as for blood culture. Sometimes procedures other than bacteriologic ones have to be performed on the specimen. In such cases centrifuge the specimen vigorously for 10 min and use the sediment for

inoculation. In interpreting the results, remember that the isolation of a few colonies in pure culture may be significant.

3. *Ear culture*. Collect the specimen with a dry, sterile cotton swab and inoculate directly onto solid media. Smear preparations should be made. Examine smears for both bacteria and fungi.

4. *Eye culture*. Collect the specimen as in ear cultures, using a fine-tipped cotton swab. Plate the specimen as soon as possible after collection. Many bacteriologically negative results obtained with eye cultures are the result of the bacteria's drying on the swab before plating.

5. *Fecal culture*. Clean around the anus; moisten a cotton swab in thioglycolate broth and insert it into the rectum. Select purulent or bloody portions from the swab for inoculation onto blood and MacConkey agar plates. When *Salmonella* spp. is suspected as the causal agent, take repeated fecal samples during the course of a day, because a negative result on one sample cultivated on a solid medium is not conclusive. In this case, rather than using swabs, collect a large fecal specimen from the rectum by digital manipulation. To encourage the selective growth of *Salmonella*, inoculate the fecal material into Selenite-F broth or tetrathionate broth. Recommended quantities are 30 g of feces into 100 ml of broth. After 6–18 hr of incubation in the selected broth, inoculate the specimen onto MacConkey agar plates and incubate at 37°C for 24 hr.

6. *Milk culture*. Collect midstream milk samples from each teat into sterile vials, inoculate onto blood and MacConkey agar plates, and incubate in both aerobic and microaerophilic environments. Examine smear preparations for bacteria and white blood cells.

7. *Necropsy culture*. Contrary to widely publicized opinions, meaningful cultures of common pathogens causing sudden death can be obtained from organs up to 24 hr after death. Whether or not meaningful cultures are obtained depends primarily on the environmental temperature after the death of the animal and the proficiency of the pathologist in collecting the specimen. Necropsy is performed in the usual manner. Before an organ or tissue is sampled, sear the surface. With a sterile pipette, enter the organ or tissue and aspirate the desired quantity of material. If possible, inoculate solid media immediately; if this is not possible, seal the open ends of the pipette in a flame and then transport or mail it to a laboratory. Another method that may be used when a culture cannot be made in a reasonable amount of time is to cut a block of tissue and store it in foil, waxed paper, or a plastic bag. At

the laboratory sear the surfaces and plate uncontaminated material from the center of the block directly onto agar plates. With small laboratory animals sterile necropsy is the preferred procedure. Samples for culture may then be taken directly from organs or tissues.

8. *Serous cavity fluid culture.* Make a smear preparation, stain it, and examine it for cells, bacteria, and fungi. Culture as for cerebrospinal fluid.

9. *Throat culture.* Wipe a dry, sterile cotton swab directly onto tonsil surface and into crypts. Inoculate onto blood and MacConkey agar plates.

10. *Urine culture.* The best specimen is one collected by cystocentesis. With a properly collected specimen, the ideal procedure is to inoculate 0.1 to 0.5 ml of urine into 8 to 10 ml of thioglycolate broth, incubate for 24 hr, and then plate onto blood and MacConkey agar and incubate aerobically and anaerobically. Broth cultures from midstream urine samples are invariably overgrown by contaminants; if the specimen is collected in this way, make heavy inoculation directly onto solid media and incubate aerobically and anaerobically.

11. *Genital culture.* When investigating reproductive problems in living female animals, introduce a dry swab of appropriate length into the cervix or neck of the uterus with the help of a speculum. In dead animals aspirate material directly from the uterus or placental membranes, inoculate the sample directly onto blood and MacConkey agar plates, and incubate in aerobic and microaerophilic environments.

12. *Wound culture.* Examine smear preparations for bacteria, fungi, and cell morphology. Inoculate routine culture media and incubate in both aerobic and anaerobic environments.

4

Direct Microscopic Examination of Specimens

1. Value in Routine Work

Direct microscopic examination of fresh unstained fecal and urine specimens can reveal useful information and can sometimes prevent the necessity of culturing. Microscopic examination of stained smear preparations can also indicate diagnosis. Often pathogenic organisms can be recognized by their shape and staining properties, together with knowledge of the host animal and site of isolation.

If an animal is undergoing a febrile reaction at the time of death, the organism will be sufficiently distributed in the blood for a smear preparation to be worthwhile. Particularly in cases of sudden death, when anthrax is a possible cause, smear preparations of blood should be examined before necropsy is performed.

Smears from cerebrospinal fluid should always be made. In most cases of listeriosis, gram-positive bacilli will be observed. A negative smear from cerebrospinal fluid should not be taken as conclusive, since occasionally only a few organisms are present, and these may not be seen but would grow as a pure culture when inoculated onto solid media.

Ear infections, particularly in dogs, can be of mycotic, parasitic, or bacterial etiology, although most are due to bacterial infection. A direct smear will show whether a multiple etiology is involved. New methylene blue or gram's stain are good general stains for ear exudates, since on these stains fungi and bacteria can be differentiated by morphology.

In general, direct examination of fecal specimens is not rewarding; however, it may indicate the presence of protozoa or parasite eggs.

When vibriosis is suspected in pigs or calves, or Johne's disease in cattle or sheep, a fecal smear preparation can be most helpful. For speed and simplicity, *Vibrio* spp. can be recognized using new methylene blue stain. When Johne's disease is suspected, the acid-fast stain for *Mycobacterium* must be used.

All mastitis milk specimens should be examined. Whether the causal organism is a *Streptococcus*, *Corynebacterium*, *Staphylococcus*, or a gram-negative bacillus can be determined readily. Occasionally no bacteria will be seen in a smear preparation, but the presence of white blood cells should be taken as an indication of mastitis. If the specimen is incubated for a few hours, organisms will be easily seen. In this system of bacteriology, a catalase test is employed. When performed on 2 ml of milk, a good bubbling reaction indicates mastitis, because white blood cells are catalase rich.

Other examples of direct examination are necropsy cultures and examination of specimens from aborted fetuses, where it is necessary to determine whether bacteria caused death. A gram-stained smear preparation can answer this question immediately. This can then be extended to presumptive recognition of the bacteria if site of isolation, host and morphology, and gram stain of the organism are known.

With cultures of urine or serous cavity fluids, the specimen must be centrifuged at 1500 rpm for 10 min. As a routine it is best to collect serous fluids into a container containing sodium EDTA (ethylenediaminetetraacetic acid). The EDTA can be put in the container first and autoclaved. Then when the specimen is collected, the EDTA is already present. Smears should be taken from the fluid or pellet in the bottom of the tube. When urine is to be examined for leptospira, darkfield examination is best. A satisfactory alternative is to make a smear and stain with Giemsa stain.

In skin wounds, if bacteria are present and are producing exotoxin, the cellular morphology will be indistinct; in the absence of exotoxin, the cellular morphology will be normal. Staphylococci produce their harmful reaction by elaborating exotoxin. Thus if a pure culture of staphylococci with normal cellular morphology is observed in a smear, it is most likely that it is a nonpathogenic strain. An example of a condition in which this occurs is interdigital cysts in dogs. In such circumstances, treatment with antibiotics or synthetic glucocorticoids is unnecessary.

If bacteria are apparent in the smear but the aerobic culture is negative, the organism is probably anaerobic.

New methylene blue stain is preferred for examining wet smear preparations of exudates.

2. Smear Preparation

Technique

1. With liquid or semisolid material, place one or two drops on a slide. Spread out to a very thin film. Air dry.
2. With feces, dilute a small portion with water and smear a thin film over the entire slide. This gives thick and thin areas and often allows clumps, particularly of acid-fast organisms, to be more readily observed. Air dry.
3. With tissue smears, gently dab a small block of tissue, held with forceps, onto the slide. Air dry.
4. With exudates, the specimen is most successfully collected with a swab. Gently roll the swab over the slide. Air dry.
5. When material is thoroughly dry, heat fix and proceed with the desired staining procedure.

3. Acid-Fast Stain

Reagents

1. Ziehl-Neelsen carbol fuchsin

   A. Dissolve 0.3 g of basic fuchsin in 10 ml of 95% ethyl alcohol.
   B. Dissolve 4.5 g of phenol in 90 ml of distilled water.

   Mix A and B. Let stand for 24 hr and filter. The solution remains stable.
2. Acid alcohol

   A. Concentrated hydrocloric acid (HCl), 2.0 ml
   B. Ethyl alcohol (95%), 98.0 ml

   Mix A and B. The solution remains stable.
3. Methylene blue stock solution

   A. Dissolve 0.5 g of methylene blue, by grinding with mortar and pestle, in a small amount of 95% ethyl alcohol. Continue adding alcohol to a total of 100 ml.
   B. Dissolve 0.01 g of potassium hydroxide in 100 ml of distilled

water. (If no analytical balance is available, prepare 100 ml of a very dilute solution)

Mix A and B. The solution remains stable for at least 12 months.

4. Methylene blue working solution

   The stock solution is usually diluted before use. One part of stock solution to nine parts of distilled water is suggested. Make fresh solution every 2 or 3 months.

Technique

1. Prepare a smear of the material to be examined. Air dry. Heat fix by passing through a flame several times.
2. Flood with carbol fuchsin and steam gently for 5 min by heating carefully with a Bunsen burner. Avoid boiling the stain. Add stain as necessary to prevent the slide from becoming dry. Wash with tap water.
3. Decolorize with acid alcohol until no more color washes out. Wash with tap water.
4. Counterstain with methylene blue for approximately 30 sec. Wash with tap water. Air dry; examine with an oil immersion objective.

Acid-fast organisms retain the red color of the initial carbol fuchsin stain. Non-acid-fast organisms lose the initial stain and take on the blue of the counterstain.

4. Dark-Field Examination

Technique

1. Place a small quantity of the material to be examined on a clean slide. Apply a clean coverslip.
2. Insert the dark-field condenser and center carefully.
3. Place a drop of immersion oil on the apex of the condenser; put the slide in position on the stage; and raise the condenser until the oil contacts the undersurface of the slide.
4. Using the low-power objective, focus the condenser by raising and lowering it until the boundary of the spot of light appears its sharpest.
5. View the slide, making slight adjustments if necessary to obtain the best detail.
6. Turn to high power and examine for motile spiraled rods.

5. Giemsa Stain

Technique

1. Make a thin smear of the material to be examined. (Urine must be centrifuged and the sediment examined.)
2. Fix in absolute methyl alcohol for several minutes.
3. Immerse in dilute Giemsa stain (1 part of stain to 19 parts of Wright's buffer is preferred) for approximately 15 min.
4. Wash with distilled water and air dry.
5. Examine for spirochetes with an oil immersion objective. Spiral-shaped organisms stain blue.

6. Gram Stain

Reagents

1. Gentian violet
   A. Dissolve 0.4 g of crystal violet (85% dye content) in 2.0 ml of 95% ethyl alcohol. Add 18.0 ml of distilled water.
   B. Dissolve 0.8 g of ammonium oxalate in 80 ml of distilled water.

   Mix A and B. The solution remains stable for a long time.
2. Gram's iodine: Dissolve 1 g of iodine and 2 g of potassium iodide in 300 ml of distilled water. Store in a dark, red-tinged glass bottle.
3. 95% ethyl alcohol
4. Safranin: Dissolve 2.5 g of safranin in 100 ml of 95% ethyl alcohol. Dilute this stock safranin solution 1 : 10 with distilled water. Store in a dark glass bottle.

Technique

1. Place a drop of water on a microscope slide.
2. Sear a small wire loop in a flame. When it is cool, pick a single colony from the culture plate and suspend it evenly in a drop of water on a slide. When several gram stains are to be done, subdivide the slide with a chinagraph pencil into 6, 8, or 10 sections and suspend a different colony in a drop of water in each square.
3. Allow the suspension of the organism to dry. Then fix it by gently heating the slide over a flame. (Passing it through the flame several times is usually adequate.)
4. For best results, set up four staining bottles (Coplin jars) containing

reagents 1, 2, 3, and 4 above; have on hand a large beaker containing clear water and a supply of paper towels.

5. Immerse the slide in gentian violet solution for at least 1 min. Rinse in water.
6. Immerse the slide in gram's iodine for at least 1 min. Rinse in tap water.
7. Decolorize by immersing in 95% ethyl alcohol for exactly 10 sec. Rinse in water.
8. Counterstain by immersing in safranin solution for at least ½ min. Rinse in water. Blot or air dry.
9. Examine the slide using an oil immersion lens.

Gram-positive organisms retain the blue of the gentian violet. Gram-negative organisms are decolorized and take on the red of the counterstain. If poor staining is observed, replace the iodine solution.

7. New Methylene Blue Stain

Reagents and Preparation

Dissolve 0.5 g of new methylene blue powder and 1.6 g of potassium oxalate in 100 ml of water. Filter before using.

Technique

1. Place a drop of new methylene blue stain on a clean glass slide.
2. Add a small amount of the material to be examined (for example, one drop of blood or one drop of urine sediment).
3. Cover with a coverslip and examine under low and high magnification.

5

Identification of Bacteria

1. Scheme for Identification

When a specimen has been cultured on blood and MacConkey agar, presumptive identification of most veterinary pathogens can be made from knowledge of (a) host animal, (b) TSI agar reaction, (c) gram stain, and (d) catalase reaction.

Figure 1 gives an overall flow diagram for the handling of a specimen for bacterial culture. Three steps are involved: (a) direct smear, (b) culture onto blood agar and MacConkey agar, and (c) culture onto selected media. Organisms requiring specialized media—for example, *Leptospira*, *Mycoplasma*, *Mycobacterium*, and *Pasteurella tularensis*—are not routinely cultivated and will not be discussed further. The decision whether microaerophilic or anaerobic culture should be made depends on the site of isolation.

Many media are available for the successful cultivation of bacteria. The following is a simple workable system that can be used by the practicing veterinarian. The specimen is cultured onto both blood agar and MacConkey agar plates unless prior incubation in broth is necessary. Cultures are observed daily for growth. A negative culture, in terms of common veterinary pathogens, is the absence of growth after three days. Blood cultures should be incubated for longer, at least seven days, before declared negative. Once growth is established, all aerobic cultures are transferred to a tube of TSI agar. Transfer is accomplished by removing a single colony from a solid medium with a straight wire rather than the conventional loop. The single colony is inoculated into the TSI agar by stabbing into the butt and streaking the slant. After 24 hr of growth in this medium the reactions are recorded. Longer incubation is rarely required. In the case of gram-positive organisms, ability to produce catalase is also tested.

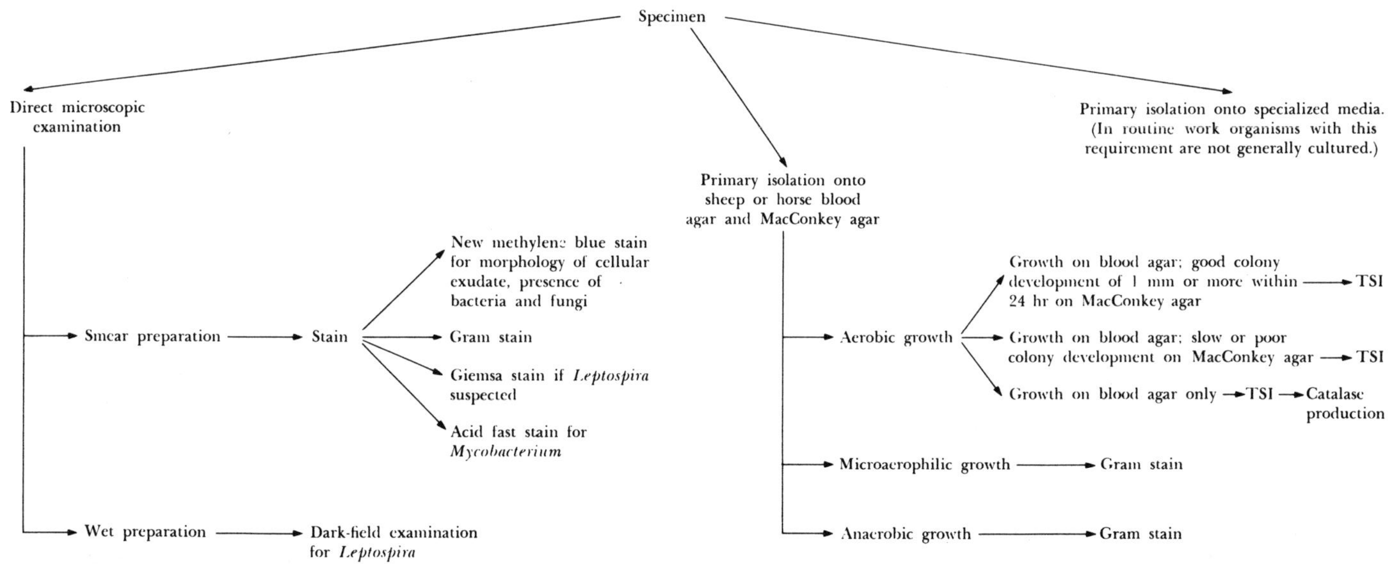

Figure 1. Flow sheet for the laboratory isolation of the more frequently occurring pathogenic bacteria.

The initial decision in this system for bacterial identification is whether growth occurs on both blood agar and MacConkey agar or on blood agar only. Organisms that grow on MacConkey agar are further subdivided into those which readily establish themselves and make obvious colony growth of 1 mm or more within 24 hr and those which take two or three days to establish themselves. This division is usually clear-cut, and presents no difficulties.

Figure 2 gives detailed steps for the presumptive recognition of the common veterinary pathogenic bacteria. Only three reactions are observed on TSI agar. (Other reactions do occur, but they are often not so clear-cut.) When H_2S is produced, the agar becomes black; this reaction is clearly positive or negative. The color of TSI agar is a pale magenta. In the presence of an organism which can fermentatively utilize glucose, the color in the butt (base) of the tube becomes a pronounced yellow. In the absence of glucose utilization, no color change occurs.

Some organisms grow on blood agar only. These are subcultured into TSI agar and gram stained. Gram-positive organisms are examined for catalase production by adding approximately 1 ml of 3% hydrogen peroxide solution to the 24-hr TSI growth. A bubbling reaction is positive.

In sum, when a smear preparation does not provide the necessary information for presumptive recognition, the specimen is cultured on a solid medium. (Exceptions are blood, cerebrospinal fluid, urine, and feces, which may, if necessary, be cultured in broth prior to plating.) The following procedure is used.

1. Inoculate by streaking MacConkey or blood agar plates and incubate at 37°C.
2. Examine daily for growth and classify as follows:
   (a) growth on MacConkey agar, rapidly growing organisms;
   (b) growth on MacConkey agar, slowly growing organisms;
   (c) growth on blood agar only, gram-negative organisms;
   (d) growth on blood agar only, gram-positive organisms.
3. Inoculate a single colony into a TSI agar tube by stabbing into the butt and streaking the slant.
4. Test gram-positive organisms for catalase production.

More specific tests than those previously presented are required to establish the identification of bacteria. The necessary tests are given in Section 2. No test in which the reaction is delayed longer than 48 hr

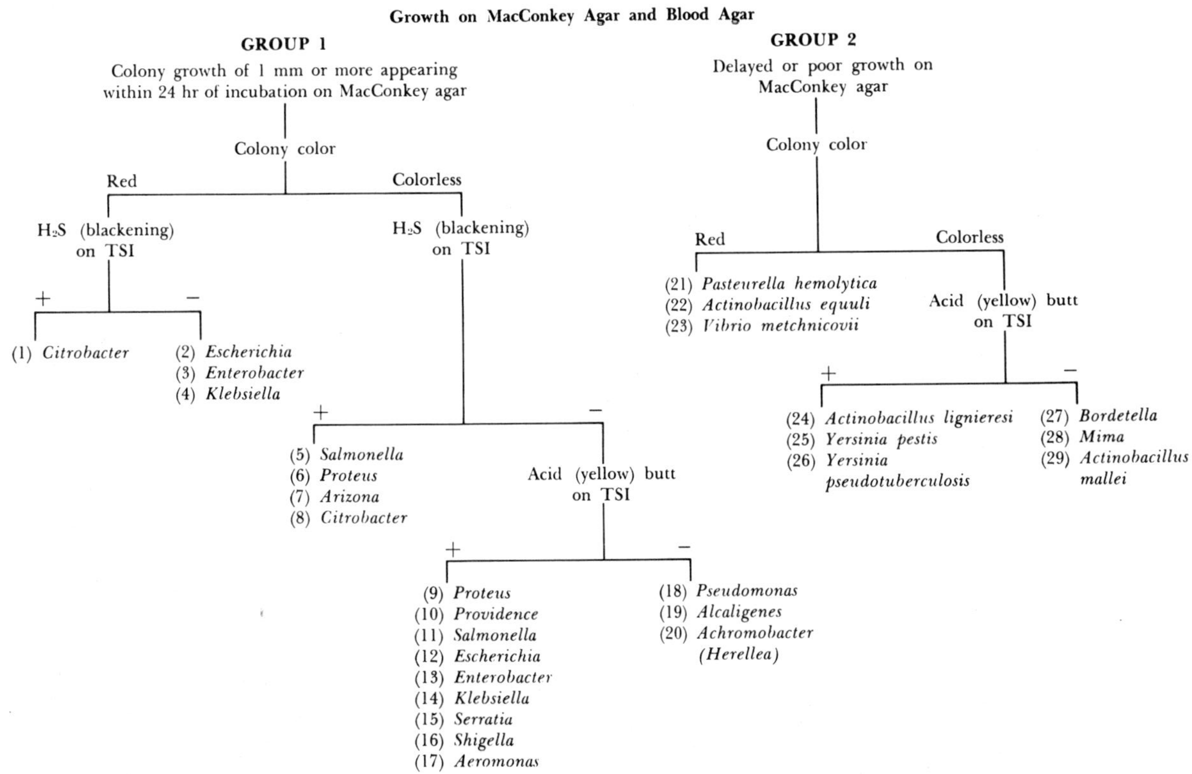

Figure 2. Outline of steps for presumptive identification of bacteria. The tests under consideration are indicated on the vertical lines, and results of the tests are on the horizontal lines directly below the tests.

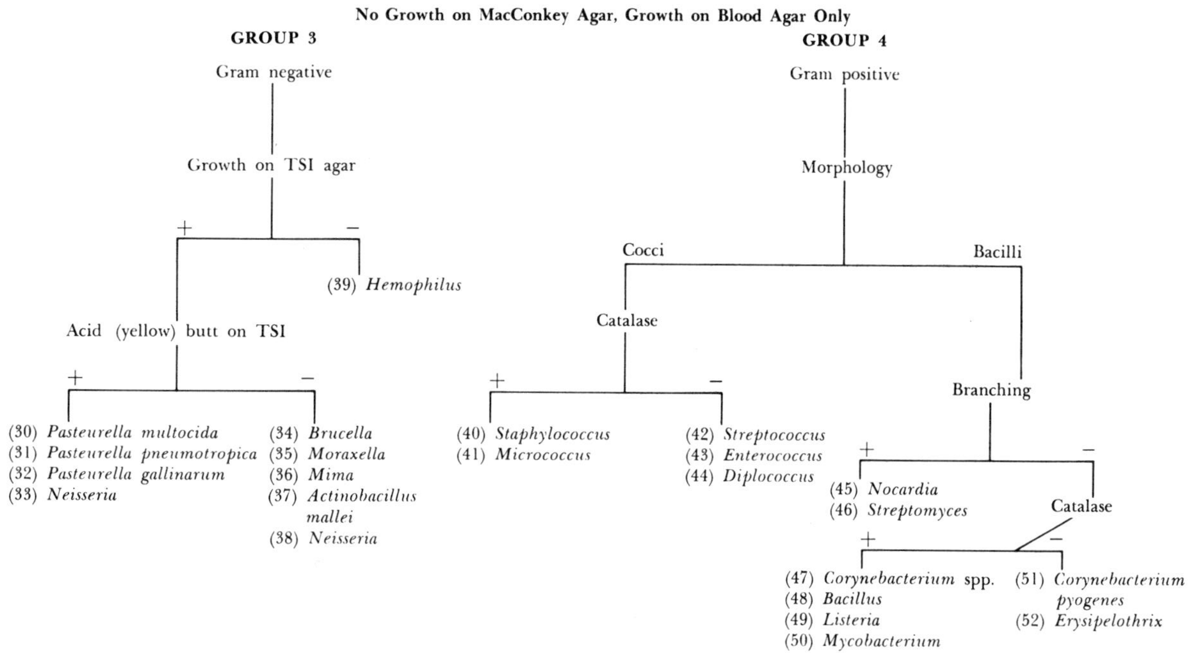

Figure 2 (Continued)

Organisms with Special Growth Requirements

GROUP 5

Special nutritional requirements

(53) *Hemophilus**
(54) *Leptospira*
(55) *Mycobacterium*
(56) *Pasteurella tularensis*
(57) *Mycoplasma*
(58) *Colesiota*
(59) *Coxiella*

GROUP 6

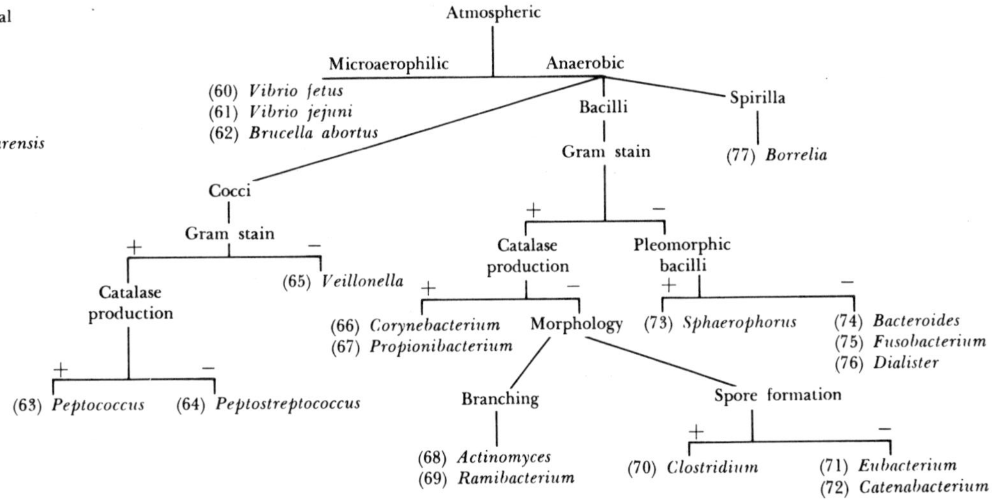

**Hemophilus* will grow on sheep or horse blood agar.

Figure 2 (Continued)

is used in this section. Each organism is numbered and these same numbers are used in the various figures 1 and 2. This enables quick and easy reference throughout the sections of this chapter.

2. Key Distinguishing Characteristics of Genera of Bacteria in Domestic Animals

Group I. Rapid Colony Development on MacConkey Agar

Group I(a). Rapid lactose fermentation (red colonies) (Table 1)

1. *Citrobacter:* H_2S production. Intestine, not usually pathogenic. No hemolysis. (*Citrobacter freundii.*)
2. *Escherichia:* Varied natural distribution, isolated more frequently from the following sites: urinary tract, intestine, udder, genitalia. Variable hemolysis. Pathogenicity based on serological characteristics. Biochemical characteristics such as hemolysis and sorbitol fermentation no longer considered as evidence for pathogenicity. (*Escherichia coli.*)
3. *Enterobacter:* Udder, intestine (intestinal strains not usually pathogenic). No hemolysis. Colonies may be confluent and slimy. Organisms produce either urease or lysine decarboxylase; they never produce both simultaneously. (*Enterobacter aerogenes, Enterobacter liquefaciens.*)

TABLE 1

	Gram stain	Citrate utilization	H_2S production (blackening on TSI)	Indole production	Motility	Urease production	Lysine decarboxylase production
*Arizona**	–		+	–	+	–	+
Citrobacter	–	+	+	v	+	v	–
Escherichia	–	–	–	+	+	–	v
Enterobacter†	–	+	–	–	+	v	v
Klebsiella	–	+	–	–	–	+	+

*Very occasionally *Arizona* ferments lactose.
†*Enterobacter* never produces both urease and lysine decarboxylase.

4. *Klebsiella:* Genitalia, udder, wounds, respiratory tract. No hemolysis. Colonies tend to be confluent and slimy. Always produce both urease and lysine decarboxylase. (*Klebsiella pneumoniae*, *Klebsiella pneumoniae* var. *genitalium*.)

Group I(b). No or delayed lactose fermentation (colorless colonies); production of H_2S (Table 2)

5. *Salmonella:* Intestine, genitalia, urinary tract. No hemolysis. (*Salmonella typhimurium*, *Salmonella anatum*, *Salmonella bredeney*, *Salmonella cholerae-suis*, *Salmonella abortus equi*, *Salmonella dublin*, *Salmonella newport*.)
6. *Proteus:* Varied natural distribution, isolated more frequently from the following sites: urinary tract, intestine, wounds. No hemolysis. 'Swarming'' over blood agar plate common. Characteristic odor. Urease production. (*Proteus mirabilis*.)
7. *Arizona:* Intestine. No hemolysis. Taxonomic position of *Arizona* group uncertain. By classical taxonomy, the *Arizona* group belongs to the genus *Salmonella*. (*Salmonella arizonae*.)
8. *Citrobacter:* as in 1.

TABLE 2

	Gram stain	Urease production	Lysine decarboxylase production	Malonate utilization	Agglutination, *Salmonella* antiserum
Salmonella	–	–	+	–	+
Proteus	–	+	–	–	–
Arizona	–	–	+	+	– (or w+)
Citrobacter	–	– (or w+)*	–	– (or w+)	–

*w+ = weak positive occasionally.

Salmonella, *Proteus*, and *Arizona* possess many common characteristics. Since *Salmonella* have significant clinical importance, to confirm identification it is necessary to examine the agglutination reaction between the organism and a commercially available polyvalent *Salmonella* antiserum.*

**Salmonella* O Antiserum, polyvalent A-I, BBL Division of Bioquest, Cockeysville, Maryland.

Group I(c). No lactose fermentation (colorless colonies); glucose fermentation (yellow butt on TSI) (Table 3)

9. *Proteus:* as in 6.
10. *Providence:* Urinary tract, intestine. No hemolysis.
11. *Salmonella:* as in 5.
12. *Escherichia:* as in 2.
13. *Enterobacter:* as in 3.
14. *Klebsiella:* as in 4.
15. *Serratia:* Urinary tract. No hemolysis, but frequently shows lysis around groups of colonies. (*Serratia marcescens.*)
16. *Shigella:* Intestine, primates. No hemolysis. (*Shigella dysenteriae, Shigella sonnei.*)
17. *Aeromonas:* Skin, tissue of fish. Beta hemolysis. (*A. salmonicida.*)

TABLE 3

	Gram stain	Urease production	Indole production	Citrate utilization	Voges–Proskauer reaction	Motility	Arabinose fermentation	Lysine decarboxylase production	Agglutination, *Salmonella* antiserum	Oxidase production
Proteus	–	+	v	v	–	+	–	–	–	–
Providence	–	–	+	+	–	+	–	–	–	–
Salmonella	–	–	–	+	–	+	+	+	+	–
Escherichia	–	–	+	–	–	+	+	v	–	–
Enterobacter	–	– (or w+)	–	+	+	+	+	v	–	–
Klebsiella	–	+	–	+	+	–	+	+	–	–
Serratia	–	w+	–	+	+	+	–	+	–	–
Shigella	–	–	–	–	–	–	v	–	–	–
Aeromonas	–	–	–	v	v	v	v	v	–	+

Group I(d). Delayed or no lactose fermentation (colorless colonies); no glucose fermentation (no change in butt on TSI agar) (Table 4)

18. *Pseudomonas:* Wounds, udder, urine, many other sites. Usually beta hemolysis, but not always evident in 24 hr. Greenish pigment common. Characteristic "fruity" odor. *Pseudomonas aeruginosa:* A nonpigmented *Pseudomonas* causes a pneumonic disease in man, resembling glanders. This disease, melioidosis, has been reported in servicemen returning from Vietnam. It has not been reported in

animals in North America. In Southeast Asia and Australia, infected cats, dogs, horses, and sheep have been reported. *Pseudomonas pseudomallei:* This organism is closely related to *Actinobacillus mallei.*

19. *Achromobacter* (*Herellea*)*:* Many sites. No hemolysis. Often diplococcoid. (*Achromobacter anitratum.*)
20. *Alcaligenes:* Urinary tract, intestine. Not considered pathogenic in the intestine. No hemolysis. (*Alcaligenes faecalis.*)

TABLE 4

	Gram stain	Oxidase production	OF glucose reaction	Motility	Nitrate reduction
P. aeruginosa	−	+	O	+	+
P. pseudomallei	−	+	F	+	+
Achromobacter	−	−	O	−	−
Alcaligenes	−	+	−	+	+(−)

Group II. Slow or Poor Colony Development on MacConkey Agar

Group II(a). Rapid lactose fermentation (red colonies) (Table 5)

21. *Pasteurella hemolytica:* Respiratory tract. Beta hemolysis.
22. *Actinobacillus equuli* (*Shigella equirulis*)*:* Genitalia, blood, intestine. Rough colony form is nonhemolytic, dry, adherent; smooth form may be beta hemolytic, moist.

TABLE 5

	Gram stain	Urease production	Motility
P. hemolytica	−	−	−
A. equuli	−	+	−
V. metschnikovii	−	−	+

23. *Vibrio metschnikovii:* Intestine. Chicken. No hemolysis. Curved and "S" forms.

Group II(b). Delayed or no lactose fermentation (colorless colonies); glucose fermentation (yellow butt on TSI) (Table 6)

24. *Actinobacillus lignieresi:* Caseous abscesses, especially of the sub-

TABLE 6

	Gram stain	Oxidase production	Urease production	Motility	Hemolysis on blood agar
A. lignieresi	–	+	+	–	v
Y. pestis	–	–	–	–	–
Y. pseudotuberculosis	–	–	+	+	–
*Pasteurella hemolytica**	–	+	–	–	+
Vibrio comma†	–	+	–	+	–

*Late lactose fermentation may result in colorless colonies on MacConkey agar.
†Usually requires CO_2 for initial isolation.

TABLE 7

	Gram stain	Oxidase production	Urease production	Motility	Diplococcoid morphology	Indole production	Nitrate reduction
Bordetella	–	+	+	+	–	–	+
Mima	–	–*	–	–	+	–	–
A. mallei	–	–	–	–	–	–	+
Rare isolates							
Vibrio fetus	–	+	–	+	–	–	+
Brucella abortus†							
Type I	–	+	+	–	–	–	+
Moraxella sp.							
Type II	–	+	+	–	+	–	+(–)
Flavobacterium	–	+	–	–	–	+	–

*Occasionally positive; known as *Mima polymorpha* var. *oxidans*.
†Usually requires CO_2 for initial isolation; *Brucella abortus* (Type I) is also penicillin resistant.

maxillary lymph nodes. "Sulfur granules" consist of uniform gram-negative bacilli. Growth improved in CO_2 rich atmosphere. No hemolysis.

25. *Yersinia* (*Pasteurella*) *pestis:* Tissues. Rodents. No hemolysis.
26. *Yersinia* (*Pasteurella*) *pseudotuberculosis:* Caseous necrotic lesions. Needs temperature below 30°C. No hemolysis.

Group II(c). Delayed or no lactose fermentation (colorless colonies); no glucose fermentation (no change in butt on TSI agar) (Table 7)

27. *Bordetella:* Respiratory tract. Beta hemolysis. (*Bordetella bronchiseptica.*)
28. *Mima:* Varied natural distribution. No hemolysis. (*Mima polymorpha.*)
29. *Actinobacillus* (*Malleomyces*) *mallei:* Respiratory tract, skin. No hemolysis. Slender bacilli. Only few strains grow on MacConkey agar; most react as in 37.

Group III. Growth on Blood Agar but no Growth on MacConkey Agar; Organisms Gram Negative

Group III(a). Glucose fermentation (yellow butt on TSI) (Table 8)

30. *Pasteurella multocida:* Wounds, respiratory tract, udder. No hemolysis. Musty odor.
31. *Pasteurella pneumotropica:* Respiratory tract. Rodent. No hemolysis.
32. *Pasteurella gallinarum:* Respiratory tract, intestine. Chicken.

TABLE 8

	Gram stain	Urease production	Indole production	Nitrate reduction	Diplococcoid morphology	Oxidase production
*P. multocida**	−	−	+	+	−	+
P. pneumotropica†	−	+	+	+	−	+
P. gallinarum	−	−	−	−	−	+
Neisseria	−	−	−	−	+	+

*Key reactions of *Pasteurella multocida* are those involving indole and nitrate.
†May need a drop of serum on slant to give positive urease production.

33. *Neisseria:* Many sites. No hemolysis. Cocci, often kidney shaped, and appearing in pairs with the flat sides adjacent. Only few strains show this reaction; most react as in 38. (*Neisseria catarrhalis.*)

Group III(b). No glucose fermentation (no change in butt on TSI agar) (Table 9)

34. *Brucella:* Genitalia, udder. Growth improved in CO_2 atmosphere. *Brucella melitensis*, *Brucella canis*, and *Brucella suis* grow in air; *Brucella abortus* and *Brucella bovis* are strict microaerophils. No hemolysis; tiny coccobacilli. (*Brucella abortus* Type I is discussed in Group II(c); *Brucella abortus* which will not grow on MacConkey agar is penicillin sensitive and is known as *Brucella abortus* Type II.)
35. *Moraxella:* Eye. Beta hemolysis. Gram negative but irregular decolorization and some appear gram positive. (*Moraxella bovis.*) The specific name of the organism causing conjunctivitis in cats has not been established (*Moraxella* spp.)
36. *Mima:* Most strains show reactions as in 28.
37. *Actinobacillus mallei:* Most strains grow on blood agar only; refer to 29. There is a close antigenic relationship between *Actinobacillus mallei* and *Pseudomonas pseudomallei*.
38. *Neisseria:* These are the common reactions for this organism; refer to 33.

TABLE 9

	Gram stain	Morphology	Oxidase production	Urease production	Beta hemolysis	Motility
Brucella	–	bacillus	+	+	–	–
Moraxella	–	diplococcoid	+	–	+	–
Mima	–	diplococcoid	– (rarely +)	– (rarely +)	–	–
A. mallei	–	bacillus	–	–	–	–
P. pseudomallei	–	bacillus	+		–	+
Neisseria	–	diplococcus	+	–	–	–

Group III(c). No growth on TSI

39. *Hemophilus:* Respiratory tract and genitalia. Variable hemolysis.

If not cultivated on horse or sheep blood agar, additional growth factors required. (Heating blood agar to 70–75°C until it turns brown, before pouring the agar into petri dishes, provides the X-factor; growing *Staphylococcus* provides the diphosphopyridine nucleotide, the V-factor.) Probably parasitic rather than pathogenic. (*Hemophilus canis*, *Hemophilus bovis*, *Hemophilus ovis*, *Hemophilus suis*.) Commercial strips (Taxo Strips, BBL) are available on which X- and V-factors have been impregnated.

Group IV. Growth on Blood Agar but no Growth on MacConkey Agar; Organisms Gram Positive

Group IV(a). Gram-positive, catalase-producing cocci (Table 10)

40. *Staphylococcus:* Varied natural distribution; isolated more frequently from the following sites: wounds, abscesses, udder, and genitalia. Variable hemolysis. White to yellow colonies. Tend to appear as clusters of cocci. (*Staphylococcus aureus*, *Staphylococcus epidermidis*.)
41. *Micrococcus:* Varied natural distribution. Not considered pathogenic. No hemolysis. (*Micrococcus ascoformans*.)

TABLE 10

	Gram stain	Coagulase production*	Acid butt on TSI agar
S. aureus	+	+	+
S. epidermidis	+	−	+
Micrococcus	+	−	−

*Coagulase reaction should be done using homologous plasma.

Group IV(b). Gram-positive cocci; no catalase production (Tables 11 and 12)

42. *Streptococcus:* Varied natural distribution isolated more frequently from the following sites: wounds, abscesses, udder, genitalia, urinary tract, and respiratory tract. Variable hemolysis. Tiny colonies in 24 hr. Cocci often in chain formations. Streptococci were

subdivided into a large number of groups by Dr. Lancefield in 1933. Her groupings are now known as Lancefield groups A, B, C, D, E, F, G, H, K, L, M, N, and O. *Streptococcus pyogenes* is a member of Lancefield's group A. Other veterinary important streptococci belong to the other groups. (*Streptococcus pyogenes*, *Streptococcus agalactiae*, *Streptococcus equi*, *Streptococcus zoo-*

TABLE 11

	Bacitracin sensitivity	Growth in *Streptococcus faecalis* SF broth	Growth in 6.5% NaCl	Optochin sensitivity
*Streptococcus**	–	–	–	–
S. pyogenes, group A	+	–	–	–
"Enterococci," group D	–	+	+	–
Diplococcus	–	–	–	+

*All Lancefield groups of *Streptococcus* except A and D.

TABLE 12

	Lancefield group	Hemolysis	Bacitracin sensitivity	Camp test	Inulin fermentation	Lactose fermentation	Sorbitol fermentation	Salicin fermentation	Growth in SF broth	Optochin sensitivity
S. pyogenes	A	beta	+	–	–	+	–	+	–	–
S. agalactiae	B	v	–	+	–	+	–	+	–	–
S. uberis	C	v	–	+	+	+	+	+	–	–
S. dysgalactiae	C	v	–	–	–	+	v	–	–	–
S. equi	C	v	–	–	–	–	–	+	–	–
S. zooepidemicus	C	beta	–	–	–	+	+	+	–	–
S. equisimilis	C	beta	–	–	–	v	–	+	–	–
S. canis	C	beta	–	–	–	+	–	+	–	–
"Enterococci"	D	v	–	–	–	+	v	+	+	–
D. pneumoniae		alpha	–	–	+	+		v	–	+

*On horse blood agar.

epidemicus, Streptococcus equisimilis, Streptococcus dysgalactiae, Streptococcus viscolactis.)

43. "Enterococci": Group D *Streptococcus* are frequently called "enterococci" or "fecal strepts." Intestine, urinary tract. Variable hemolysis. Cocci often in lancet arrangement. (*Streptococcus faecalis, Streptococcus durans, Streptococcus liquefaciens.*)
44. *Diplococcus:* Respiratory tract. Alpha hemolysis. Tiny colonies in 24 hr. Pairs of cocci often in lancet arrangement. (*Diplococcus pneumoniae.*)

Group IV(c). Gram-positive bacilli (Tables 13, 14, and 15)

45. *Nocardia:* Exudates from granulomatous lesions of a variety of tissues; frequently from lungs and lymph nodes. Direct smear of "sulfur granules" shows gram-positive, partially acid-fast, branching filaments. Slow aerobic growth. No hemolysis. Sometimes classified as a fungus. (*Nocardia asteroides, Nocardia farcinica*)
46. *Streptomyces:* Fungus widely distributed in nature. Difficult to distinguish morphologically from *Nocardia*. Nonpathogenic contaminant.
47. *Corynebacterium* spp.: Varied natural distribution, isolated most frequently from the following sites: genitalia, abscesses. Many are nonpathogenic. Usually not hemolytic; pleomorphic coccobacilli. (*Corynebacterium renale, Corynebacterium equi,* and *Corynebacterium ovis.*)

TABLE 13

Branching organisms	"Sulfur granules" in pathological material	Production of aerial mycelium and conidia	Casein hydrolysis†	Production of tyrosinase
Nocardia sp.*	+	–	–	–
Streptomyces sp.	–	+	+	+

*May be weakly acid-fast.
†Within three days.

TABLE 14

Gram-positive bacilli	Beta hemolysis	Acid-fast	H_2S on TSI agar	Motility	Spore formation
Corynebacterium spp.	−(+)	−	−	−	−
Bacillus sp.	+(−)	−	−	+	+
B. anthracis	−	−	−	−	+
Listeria	+	−	−	+†	−
Mycobacterium	−	+	−	−	−
C. pyogenes	+	−	−	−	−
Erysipelothrix	−(+)	−	+*	−	−

*May take from three to five days for blackening to become evident.
†Best demonstrated at room temperature.

48. *Bacillus:* Many strains, usually not pathogenic. Variable hemolysis, usually motile. *Bacillus anthracis* is a highly pathogenic member of this genus. It may be isolated from blood, tissues. No hemolysis, nonmotile; long chains of square-ended bacilli on blood agar.
49. *Listeria:* Placenta, brain, blood, and udder. Refrigerating specimen several weeks may aid isolation. Beta hemolysis, tumbling motility at room temperature. May appear as cocci. (*Listeria monocytogenes*)
50. *Mycobacterium:* Lung, abscesses, bone, intestine. Direct smear of caseous material or intestinal mucosa shows slender, beaded acid-fast bacilli, often in clumps. Slow growth on blood agar, no hemolysis. Special media preferred. Candle jar may aid growth. (*Mycobacterium tuberculosis*, *Mycobacterium bovis*, *Mycobacterium paratuberculosis*.) *Mycobacterium paratuberculosis* is difficult to cultivate and requires up to six weeks for colony growth. Therefore it is best to diagnose Johne's disease by the presence of acid-fast bacilli from feces or intestinal content.
51. *Corynebacterium pyogenes:* Wounds, abscesses, genitalia. Beta hemolysis, with the colonies often not visible until a day or two after hemolysis is seen. Pleomorphic coccobacilli with "palisading" a common feature.
52. *Erysipelothrix:* Tissues, blood. Slow growth, candle jar incubation preferred. Weak alpha to beta hemolysis. Slender bacilli. Slow

H_2S production on TSI agar, often not evident for three or four days. *Erysipelothrix insidiosa:* Smooth form: slender rods. Colonies pinpoint, colorless, glistening. Rough form: long filamentous, branching, beading, swelling. Colonies larger, granular curled appearance (like miniature *Bacillus anthracis*).

TABLE 15

Corynebacterium	Hemolysis	Catalase production	Acid butt in TSI glucose fermentation	Lactose fermentation	Sucrose fermentation
C. pyogenes	+	−	+	+	+
C. equi	−	+	−	−	−
C. renale	−(+)	+	+	−	−
C. pseudotuberculosis	−(+)	+	+	+	+

Group V. Organisms with Special Nutritional Requirements

53. *Hemophilus:* Respiratory tract and genitalia. Variable hemolysis. If not cultivated on horse or sheep blood agar, additional growth factors are required. (Heating blood agar to 70°–75°C until it turns brown, before pouring the agar into petri dishes, provides the X-factor; growing *Staphylococcus* provides the diphosphopyridine nucleotide, the V-factor.) Probably parasitic rather than pathogenic. (*Hemophilus canis*, *Hemophilus bovis*, *Hemophilus ovis*, *Hemophilus suis*.)
54. *Leptospira:* Tissues, blood, urinary tract, abscesses. Motile, spiraled rods, best viewed by dark-field illumination; may be stained by Giemsa stain. Commercially prepared media are available for culture. (*Leptospira canicola*, *Leptospira icterohaemorrhagiae*, *Leptospira grippotyphosa*, *Leptospira bovis*, *Leptospira pomona*, *Leptospira sejroe*.)
55. *Mycobacterium:* as in 49.
56. *Pasteurella tularensis:* Tissues, blood. Rabbits, rodents. Requires cystine in culture media; slow growth; often causes a green discoloration of blood; tiny coccobacilli, often pleomorphic.
57. *Mycoplasma:* Respiratory tract, many other sites. Some strains grow on blood agar, often hemolytic. Various enrichments assist

growth of the more fastidious species. Colonies may be barely visible even after long incubation. Pleomorphic, ring forms, filaments. Not stained by Gram stain; use Giemsa or new methylene blue; very pleomorphic. (*Mycoplasma agalactiae*, *Mycoplasma mycoides*, *Mycoplasma hyorhinis* and *Mycoplasma hyopneumoniae*.)

58. *Colesiota:* Eye, sheep. Organism belongs to the order Rickettsiales. Requires specialized equipment for artificial cultivation. Gram negative. (*Colesiota conjunctivae*.)
59. *Coxiella:* Blood tissues; organism belongs to order Rickettsiales. Pleomorphic, varying in size from pinpoint to short rod. (*Coxiella burneti*.)

Group VI(a). Microaerophilic environment

60. *Vibrio fetus:* Genitalia. Slow growth, microaerophilic atmosphere for incubation essential. Variable hemolysis. Curved and "sea gull" bacilli.
61. *Vibrio:* Intestine. Slow growth, microaerophilic atmosphere for incubation preferred. Variable hemolysis. Curved and "sea gull" bacilli. Differentiate from *Vibrio fetus* by site of isolation. (*Vibrio coli*, *Vibrio jejuni*.)
62. *Brucella:* Genitalia, udder. Microaerophilic atmosphere incubation preferred. (*Brucella abortus* and *Brucella suis* are obligate microaerophiles on initial isolation.) No hemolysis. Tiny coccobacilli.

Group VI(b). Anaerobic environment

63. *Peptococcus:* Wounds, urinary tract. Gram-positive, catalase-positive cocci. Usually not hemolytic. (*Peptococcus asaccharolyticus*.)
64. *Peptostreptococcus:* Wounds, abscesses, fistulae, urinary tract. Anaerobic conditions required for initial isolation. Alpha or beta hemolysis. Gram-positive, catalase-negative cocci usually appearing in long chains; colonies may be subsurface. (*Peptostreptococcus anaerobius*.)
65. *Veillonella:* Intestine. Strict anaerobic gram-positive cocci appearing as pairs, chains, or masses. Do not reduce nitrates or produce indole; no attack on carbohydrates; not known to be pathogenic to animals. (*Veillonella alcalescens*; *Veillonella parvula*.)
66. *Corynebacterium:* Skin inhabitants of most animals; isolated from urine and wounds in domestic animals. Gram positive, pleo-

morphic. Very slow growing, requiring up to one week for colony development. Liquify gelatin and reduce nitrates. (*Corynebacterium acnes.*)

67. *Propionibacterium:* Isolated from dairy products. Nonpathogenic. Gram positive; pleomorphic; slow growing. Do not liquify gelatin or reduce nitrates.
68. *Actinomyces:* Exudates from encapsulated abscesses, frequently around mandible and tongue. Direct smear of "sulfur granules" shows gram-positive, branching filaments. Anaerobic atmosphere required for culture. Not hemolytic. Sometimes classified as fungi. (*Actinomyces bovis*; *Actinomyces baudeti.*) (Table 16)

TABLE 16

	Growth in thioglycolate broth	Morphology	Nitrate reduction	Mannitol fermentation
A. bovis	diffuse	branching rare, few filaments	–	–
A. baudeti	granular, clear broth	branching, filamentous	+	+

69. *Ramibacterium:* Wide natural distribution. Cells arranged in Y- or V-formations. Strict anaerobes. Nonmotile. Produce gas in thioglycolate broth. (*Ramibacterium ramosoides*; *Ramibacterium ramosum.*)
70. *Clostridium:* Tissues, wounds, blood, intestine. Anaerobic atmosphere required for culture. Beta hemolysis common. Medium to large gram-positive bacilli, appearing singly and in chains; nearly all acidify the butt on TSI agar and produce gas. Catalase negative. Form spores. In the clinical laboratory, precise separation of Clostridia is time consuming. Normally check for the Clostridia which is suspected. It has been our experience that some tests, such as proteolysis or the reaction on litmus milk, take a long time (up to 14 days) and may not have clear end results. These tests are often recommended but are not always desirable for routine work. *Clostridium hemolyticum* will grow on blood agar only when freshly prepared. (*Clostridium novyi*, *Clostridium perfringens*,

TABLE 17

Some Typical Reactions of Clostridia

Test	*C. movyi*	*C. perfringens*	*C. septicum*	*C. hemolyticum*	*C. chauvoei*	*C. tetani*	*C. botulinum*	*C. bifermentans*	*C. tertium*	*C. sporogenes*	*C. histolyticum*
Motility	+	−	+	+	+	+	+	+	+	+	+
Glucose fermentation	+	+	+	+	+	−	+	+	+	+	−
Lactose fermentation	−	+	+	−	+	−	−	−	+	−	−
Sucrose fermentation	−	+	−	−	+	−	−	−	+	−	−
Salicin fermentation	−	−	+	−	−	−	−	+	−	−	−
Indole production	−	−	−	+	−	−	−	+	−	−	−
Nitrate reduction	−	+	+	−	+	−	−	−	+	+	−
Sulfide (H_2S) production	−	−	−	−	−	+	+	+	−	+	+
Proteolysis	−	−	−	−	−	−	+	+	−	+	+
Spore morphology*	ovoid E	ovoid C	ovoid E	ovoid ST	ovoid E	round T	ovoid E	ovoid E	ovoid T	ovoid E	ovoid ST

*C = central, E = eccentric, ST = Subterminal, T = terminal.

Clostridium septicum, *Clostridium hemolyticum*, *Clostridium chauvoei*, *Clostridium tetani*, *Clostridium botulinum*, *Clostridium bifermentans*, *Clostridium tertium*, *Clostridium sporogenes*, *Clostridium histolyticum*.) (Table 17)

71. *Eubacterium:* Intestine. Anaerobic atmosphere required. Gram positive, nonhemolytic bacillus. (*Eubacterium disciformans*, *Eubacterium obstii*.)
72. *Catenabacterium:* Intestine. Similar to *Eubacterium* except that *Catenabacterium* show chain formation. Pathogenic for guinea pigs and mice but not for domestic animals. (*Catenabacterium contortum*, *Catenabacterium lottii*, *Catenabacterium nigrum*.) (Table 18)

TABLE 18

	Morphology	Black colonies	Gas in culture media	Fetid odor
C. contortum	chains	−	+	−
C. lottii	chains	−	−	−
C. nigrum	chains	+	−	+
E. disciformans	small masses	−	−	−
E. obstii	single rods	−	+	+

73. *Sphaerophorus:* Necrotic lesions. Anaerobic atmosphere necessary. No hemolysis of horse or sheep cells but beta hemolysis with human and rabbit cells. Pleomorphic bacilli, often showing round "swollen" bodies. Catalase negative. Gram negative. (*Sphaerophorus necrophorus*, *Sphaerophorus nodosus*.) (Table 19)
74. *Bacteroides:* Necrotic lesions, intestine. Anaerobic atmosphere required. Rarely hemolytic. Fairly uniform gram-negative bacilli; catalase-negative or weakly positive. (*Bacteroides fragilis*, *Bacteroides girans*, *Bacteroides melaninogenicus*.) (Table 19)
75. *Fusobacterium:* Mouth and pharynx. Short, nonmotile gram-negative bacilli; majority of organisms have pointed ends, which is a characteristic feature. Strict anaerobe. (*Fusobacterium fusiforme*.) (Table 19)
76. *Dialister:* Respiratory tract, very small, nonhemolytic gram-negative bacilli. Produce indole. Nonpathogenic to domestic animals. (*Dialister pneumosintes*.) (Table 19)

77. *Borrelia:* Mouth, intestine. Anaerobic atmosphere required. It is the only spirillum which takes gram stain. Gram negative; large spirillum; motile. (*Borellia vincentii, Borellia canis.*)

TABLE 19

	Morphology	Beta hemolysis	Indole production	Fetid odor	Black colonies
S. necrophorus	pleomorphic rods	+	+	+	−
S. nodosus	pleomorphic rods	−	±	+	−
B. fragilis	blunt rods	−	−	+	−
B. melaninogenicus	coccobacilli	−	+	+	+*
F. fusiforme	long rods, pointed ends	−	−	−	−
D. pneumosintes	minute rods	−	+	−	−

*Usually takes from three to five days of incubation.

3. Recognizing Bacteria Affecting Cats, Dogs, Horses, Cattle, Sheep, and Pigs

The information in Figure 2 is often too general for convenient use by species-oriented veterinary practices. In this section we therefore present species-specific bacterial identification flow charts using the information given in Figure 2.

Flow Chart for the Recognition of Pathogenic Bacteria from Cats

1. Specimen inoculated onto sheep or horse blood agar and MacConkey agar

2. Good growth on MacConkey agar:
   - (a) Red colonies — (2) *Escherichia*
   - (b) Colorless colonies
     - Black on TSI — (5) *Salmonella*
     - Yellow butt on TSI — (9) *Proteus*; (11) *Salmonella*; (12) *Escherichia*
     - No change on TSI — (18) *Pseudomonas*

3. Delayed growth on MacConkey agar:
   (a) Red colonies — (21) *Pasteurella*
   (b) Colorless colonies
      No change on TSI — (27) *Bordetella*

4. Growth on blood agar only:
   (a) Gram-negative bacilli
      Yellow butt on TSI — (30) *Pasteurella*
      No change on TSI — (35) *Moraxella*
      No growth on TSI — (39) *Hemophilus*
   (b) Gram-positive cocci
      Catalase positive — (40) *Staphylococcus*; (41) *Micrococcus*
      Catalase negative — (42) *Streptococcus*
      Branching formation — (45) *Nocardia*
   (c) Gram-positive bacilli
      Catalase positive — (48) *Bacillus*; (50) *Mycobacterium*

5. Organisms with special nutritional requirements:
   (a) Gram-negative bacilli — (53) *Hemophilus*

6. Anaerobic organisms:
   (a) Gram-positive cocci
      Catalase positive — (63) *Peptococcus*
      Catalase negative — (64) *Peptostreptococcus*
   (b) Gram-positive bacilli
      Catalase positive — (66) *Corynebacterium*
      Branching formation — (68) *Actinomyces*
      Single bacilli — (70) *Clostridium*

Flow Chart for the Recognition of Pathogenic Bacteria from Dogs

1. Specimen inoculated onto sheep or horse blood agar and MacConkey agar

2. Growth on MacConkey agar:
   (a) Red colonies — (2) *Escherichia*; (4) *Klebsiella*
   (b) Colorless colonies
      Black on TSI — (5) *Salmonella*; (6) *Proteus*

Yellow butt on TSI	(9) *Proteus* (11) *Salmonella* (12) *Escherichia* (13) *Enterobacter* (14) *Klebsiella*
No change on TSI	(18) *Pseudomonas*
3. Delayed growth on MacConkey agar:	
(a) Red colonies	(21) *Pasteurella*
(b) Colorless colonies	
No change on TSI	(27) *Bordetella*
4. Growth on blood agar only:	
(a) Gram-negative bacilli	
Yellow butt on TSI	(30) *Pasteurella*
No change on TSI	(34) *Brucella*
(b) Gram-positive cocci	
Catalase positive	(40) *Staphylococcus*
Catalase negative	(42) *Streptococcus*
(c) Gram-positive bacilli	
Branching formation	(45) *Nocardia* (47) *Corynebacterium*
Catalase positive	(48) *Bacillus* (49) *Listeria* (50) *Mycobacterium*
5. Direct microscopic examination of urine	(54) *Leptospira*
6. Microaerophilic organisms:	
(a) Gram-negative bacilli	(62) *Brucella*
7. Anaerobic organisms:	
(a) Gram-positive cocci	
Catalase positive	(63) *Peptococcus*
Catalase negative	(64) *Peptostreptococcus*
(b) Gram-positive bacilli	
Catalase positive	(66) *Corynebacterium*
Catalase negative	(70) *Clostridium*
(c) Gram-negative bacilli	(74) *Fusobacterium*
(d) Gram-negative spirillum	(77) *Borrelia*

Flow Chart for the Recognition of Pathogenic Bacteria from Horses

1. Specimen inoculated onto sheep or horse blood agar and MacConkey agar	
2. Good growth on MacConkey agar:	
(a) Red colonies	(2) *Escherichia* (4) *Klebsiella*
(b) Colorless colonies	
Black on TSI	(5) *Salmonella* (6) *Proteus*
Yellow butt on TSI	(9) *Proteus* (11) *Salmonella* (12) *Escherichia* (14) *Klebsiella*
No change on TSI	(18) *Pseudomonas*
3. Delayed growth on MacConkey agar:	
(a) Red colonies	(22) *Actinobacillus*
(b) Colorless colonies	
No change on TSI	(27) *Bordetella* (29) *Actinobacillus mallei*
4. Growth on blood agar only:	
(a) Gram-negative bacilli	
Yellow butt on TSI	(30) *Pasteurella*
(b) Gram-positive cocci	
Catalase positive	(40) *Staphylococcus*
Catalase negative	(42) *Streptococcus*
(c) Gram-positive bacilli	
Catalase positive	(47) *Corynebacterium* (48) *Bacillus anthracis* (50) *Mycobacterium*
Catalase negative	(51) *Corynebacterium pyogenes*
5. Direct microscopic examination of urine	(54) *Leptospira*
6. Microaerophilic organisms:	
(a) Gram-negative bacilli	(62) *Brucella*

7. Anaerobic organisms:
   (a) Gram-positive cocci
      Catalase positive — (64) *Peptostreptococcus*
   (b) Gram-positive bacilli
      Branching formations — (68) *Actinomyces*
      Single bacilli — (70) *Clostridium*
   (c) Gram-negative bacilli
      Pleomorphic — (73) *Sphaerophorus*
      Single bacilli — (74) *Bacteroides*

Flow Chart for the Recognition of Pathogenic Bacteria from Cattle

1. Specimen inoculated onto sheep or horse blood agar and MacConkey agar

2. Good growth on MacConkey agar:
   (a) Red colonies — (2) *Escherichia*
   (b) Colorless colonies
      Black on TSI — (5) *Salmonella*, (6) *Proteus*, (7) *Arizona*
      Yellow butt on TSI — (9) *Proteus*, (11) *Salmonella*, (12) *Escherichia*, (13) *Enterobacter*, (14) *Klebsiella*
      No change on TSI — (18) *Pseudomonas*, (19) *Alcalcigenes*

3. Delayed growth on MacConkey agar:
   (a) Red colonies — (21) *Pasteurella*
   (b) Colorless colonies
      Yellow butt on TSI — (24) *Actinobacillus*, (26) *Yersinia*

4. Growth on blood agar only:
   (a) Gram-negative bacilli
      Yellow butt on TSI — (30) *Pasteurella*
      No change on TSI — (35) *Moraxella*
      No growth on TSI — (39) *Hemophilus*
   (b) Gram-positive cocci
      Catalase positive — (40) *Staphylococcus*

Catalase negative	(42) *Streptococcus*
	(44) *Diplococcus*
Branching formation	(45) *Nocardia*
(c) Gram-positive bacilli	
Catalase positive	(48) *Bacillus anthracis*
	(49) *Listeria*
	(50) *Mycobacterium*
Catalase negative	(51) *Corynebacterium pyogenes*
	(52) *Erysipelothrix*
5. Direct microscopic examination of urine	(54) *Leptospira*
6. Microaerophilic organisms:	
(a) Gram-negative comma-shaped rods	(60) *Vibrio*
(b) Gram-negative bacilli	(62) *Brucella*
7. Anaerobic organisms:	
(a) Gram-positive bacilli	
Branching formation	(68) *Actinomyces*
Single bacilli	(70) *Clostridium*
(b) Gram-negative bacilli	
Pleomorphic	(73) *Sphaerophorus*

Flow Chart for the Recognition of Pathogenic Bacteria from Sheep

1. Specimen inoculated onto sheep or horse blood agar and MacConkey agar

2. Good growth on MacConkey agar:	
(a) Red colonies	(2) *Escherichia*
	(3) *Enterobacter*
	(4) *Klebsiella*
(b) Colorless colonies	
Black on TSI	(5) *Salmonella*
	(6) *Proteus*
	(7) *Arizona*
Yellow butt on TSI	(9) *Proteus*
	(12) *Escherichia*
	(13) *Enterobacter*
	(14) *Klebsiella*

No change on TSI	(18) *Pseudomonas*
	(20) *Achromobacter*

3. Delayed growth on MacConkey agar:

(a) Red colonies	(21) *Pasteurella hemolytica*
(b) Colorless colonies	
Yellow butt on TSI	(24) *Actinobacillus ligneresi*

4. Growth on blood agar only:

(a) Gram-negative bacilli	
Yellow butt on TSI	(30) *Pasteurella*
No change on TSI	(34) *Brucella*
(b) Gram-positive cocci	
Catalase positive	(40) *Staphylococcus*
Catalase negative	(42) *Streptococcus*
	(43) *Enterococcus*
(c) Gram-positive bacilli	
Catalase positive	(47) *Corynebacterium*
	(48) *Bacillus anthracis*
	(49) *Listeria*
	(50) *Mycobacterium*
Catalase negative	(51) *Corynebacterium pyogenes*
	(52) *Erysiphelothrix*

5. Special nutritional requirement	(56) *Pasteurella pseudotuberculosis*
	(57) *Mycoplasma*
	(58) *Colesiota*

6. Microaerophilic organisms:

(a) Gram-negative comma-shaped rods	(60) *Vibrio fetus*
	(61) *Vibrio jejuni*
(b) Gram-negative bacilli	(62) *Brucella*

7. Anaerobic organisms

(a) Gram-positive bacilli	(70) *Clostridium*
(b) Gram-negative bacilli	
Pleomorphic	(73) *Sphaerophorus*

Flow Chart for the Recognition of Pathogenic Bacteria from Pigs

1. Specimen inoculated onto sheep or horse blood agar and MacConkey agar

2. Good growth on MacConkey agar:	
(a) Red colonies	(2) *Escherichia*
(b) Colorless colonies	
Black on TSI	(5) *Salmonella*
	(6) *Proteus*
Yellow butt on TSI	(9) *Proteus*
	(11) *Salmonella*
	(12) *Escherichia*
No change on TSI	(18) *Pseudomonas*
	(20) *Achromobacter*
3. Delayed growth on MacConkey agar:	
(a) Red colonies	(21) *Pasteurella*
(b) Colorless colonies	
Yellow butt on TSI	(24) *Actinobacillus*
No change on TSI	(27) *Bordetella*
4. Growth on blood agar only:	
(a) Gram-negative bacilli	
Yellow butt on TSI	(30) *Pasteurella*
No change on TSI	(34) *Brucella*
No growth on TSI	(39) *Hemophilus*
(b) Gram-positive cocci	
Catalase positive	(40) *Staphylococcus*
Catalase negative	(42) *Streptococcus*
	(47) *Corynebacterium*
	(48) *Bacillus anthracis*
(c) Gram-positive bacilli	
Catalase positive	(49) *Listeria*
Catalase negative	(51) *Corynebacterium pyogenes*
	(52) *Erysiphelothrix*
5. Direct microscopic examination of urine	(54) *Leptospira*
6. Organisms with special growth requirements	(57) *Mycoplasma*
7. Microaerophilic organisms:	
(a) Gram-negative comma-shaped rods	(61) *Vibrio*

(b) Gram-negative bacilli (59) *Brucella*

8. Anaerobic organisms:
   (a) Gram-positive bacilli
   Branching formation (68) *Actinomyces*
   (b) Gram-negative bacilli
   Pleomorphic (73) *Sphaerophorus*

4. Sterility Control and Disinfection

It is essential to prevent the environment from becoming unduly contaminated with bacteria. In the absence of sterility control and good disinfecting procedures, reliable work is impossible. The following procedures should be followed to minimize contamination:

1. At the end of a work session, sponge the bench surfaces liberally with disinfectant and leave to dry.
2. Put all used culture plates and tubes, when no longer needed, in a metal bin with a tightly fitting lid for storage. Before disposal, autoclave the cultures.
3. Clean up any spills or accidents and disinfect the area immediately.
4. Heat bacteriology loops and forceps in a Bunsen flame before and after use.
5. Do not allow animals in the laboratory area.

6

Equipment and Reagents

1. Design Features of a Modest Laboratory

The ideal practicing laboratory should have the following features:

bright clean room with good lighting and washable floors;
limited traffic pattern;
good ventilation;
benches with smooth surfaces for easy disinfection;
gas and electric outlets;
sink unit with draining board;
storage space, large cupboards, drawers of different sizes;
convenient access to incubator, stove, and refrigerator.

2. Equipment and Materials

A list of essential equipment and materials is given below. Major items are microscope, autoclave, refrigerator, and incubator. Autoclaves are expensive and must be installed by a plumber; they are therefore permanent fixtures. A most satisfactory alternative is a large (21-qt) canning pressure cooker. It is much less expensive and is more convenient to use and install. A laboratory incubator with precise temperature control is ideal, but it is a large capital item. A simple incubator, provided it can be sterilized and has a reasonably good thermostat, is quite satisfactory. Temperature should not fluctuate below 33°C or above 40°C.

Essential Equipment and Materials

* Microscope
* Incubator
* Bunsen burner
* Inoculating needle holders, needles, and loops
* Forceps
* Sensitivity disc dispenser
* Large conical flasks for medium preparation; convenient size is 1-liter capacity
* Coplin jars for holding stains
* Pipetting syringe for dispensing media (e.g., BD Cornwall pipetting syringe)
* Racks for holding culture tubes
* Disinfectant (e.g., Roccal or Amphyl)
* Microscope slides
* Cotton-tipped applicator sticks
† Pressure cooker
† Refrigerator
† Small metal rubbish bin with lid
† Waste paper basket
† Paper towel rack
Large bottles for anaerobic and microaerophilic studies

3. Media and Reagents

In this scheme of clinical bacteriology only essential media and materials are suggested. Blood agar plates, MacConkey agar plates, thioglycolate broth tubes, TSI agar slants, gram stain reagents, *Salmonella* polyvalent antiserum—all of which are readily available from laboratory supply houses—are required. A 3% solution of hydrogen peroxide is also necessary. This can be prepared by diluting one part of pharmaceutical grade hydrogen peroxide with 10 parts of water.

In Table 20 the media and reagents for the complete system are listed. Catalogue numbers of products supplied by three companies are given only because the author has always dealt with these firms and has no experience with others.

*Can be purchased from a laboratory supply house.
†Can be purchased from a department store.

TABLE 20

Source of Media and Reagents

	Item	Catalogue number	Company
Media	Agar agar	11847	BBL Division of BioQuest*
	Cysteine trypticase agar (CTA)	11096	
	Cysteine heart agar	11137	
	Fletcher medium base	11255	
	Indole nitrite medium	11298	
	Leptospira enrichment	11883	
	Lowenstein-Jenson medium base	11358	
	MacConkey medium base	11387	
	Malonite broth, Ewing modified	11398	
	Moeller decarboxylase broth base	11429	
	Mycoplasma agar base	11456	
	OF basal medium	11483	
	Petragnani medium	21121	
	Phenylethyl alcohol agar	11538	
	Cooked meat phytone medium	11129	
	Selenite-F broth	11608	
	Selenite cysteine broth	11605	
	SF broth	1157	
	SIM media	11578	
	Simmon citrate agar	11619	
	Stuart broth base	11667	
	Tetrathionate broth base	11706	
	Thioglycolate medium, fluid, without dextrose	11725	
	TSI agar	11749	
	Trypticase soy agar	11042	
	Trypticase soy broth	11767	
	Urea agar base	11794	
	Salmonella O polyvalent antisera	40707	
	Skim milk powder	11914	
	Taxo A discs	31040	
	Taxo arabinose discs	31059	
	Taxo dextrose discs	31061	
	Taxo inulin discs	31069	
	Taxo mannitol discs	31077	

(*Cont'd*)

*Address: Cockeysville, Maryland. Another manufacturer of similar products is Difco Laboratories, Detroit, Michigan.

TABLE 20 (*Continued*)

	Item	Catalogue number	Company
Media—*Cont'd*	Taxo P discs	31046	
	Taxo salicin discs	31093	
	Taxo sorbitol discs	31096	
	Taxo sucrose discs	31098	
	Yeast extract	11929	
Prepared plated media	MacConkey agar	21172	BBL Division of BioQuest*
	Phenylethyl alcohol agar	21179	
	Trypticase soy agar	21185	
	Trypticase soy agar with 5% sheep blood	21239	
Prepared tubed media	Cooked meat phytone medium	20868	BBL Division of BioQuest*
	CTA medium with dextrose	20848	
	CTA medium with lactose	20850	
	CTA medium with mannitol	20854	
	CTA medium with salicin	20856	
	CTA medium with sorbitol	20858	
	CTA medium with sucrose	20860	
	Indole nitrite medium	20890	
	Lowenstein-Jenson medium slants	20908	
	Malonate broth, Ewing modified	21322	
	Moeller decarboxylase broth with lysine	21253	
	Moeller decarboxylase broth with ornithine	21255	
	MR-VP broth	20954	
	OF medium with dextrose	21328	
	Petragnani medium slants	20976	
	SF broth	21008	
	SIM medium	21010	
	Selenite-F broth	21020	
	Simmon citrate agar slants	21026	
	TSI agar slants	21038	
	Trypticase soy broth	21092	
	Urea agar slants, complete	21096	

*Address: Cockeysville, Maryland. Another manufacturer of similar products is Difco Laboratories, Detroit, Michigan.

TABLE 20 (*Continued*)

	Item	Catalogue number	Company
Sugars	Arabinose	11961	BBL Division of BioQuest*
	Dextrose	11863	
	Inulin	12016	
	Mannitol	12023	
	Salicin	12072	
	Sorbitol	12083	
Stains	Gentian violet solution	So-G-18	Fisher Scientific†
	Iodine solution	So-I-96	
	Safranin solution	So-S-2	
	New methylene blue solution	Na-488	
	Giemsa stain	So-G-28	
	Buffer solution	So-B-122	
	Ziehl-Neelsen carbol-fuschin stain	So-c-34	
	Ferric chloride	i-88	
	Sodium sulfite	S-430	
	Methylene blue	M-291	
Chemicals	L-Lysine	L5501	Sigma Chemical Co.†
	L-Ornithine	O2375	
	Acetic acid	A-37	Fisher Scientific†
	Ammonium oxalate	A-679	
	p-Aminodimethylalanine oxalate	5672	
	Citric acid	A-940	
	Creatine	C-523	
	p-Dimethylamino-benzaldehyde	So-D-44	
	Ethyl alcohol	A-407	
	Hydrochloric acid	A-144	
	Iodine crystals	I-37	
	1-Naphthol	N-12	
	1-Naphthylamine	N-23	
	Phenol	A-931	
	Potassium hydroxide	P-250	
	Potassium iodide	P-257	
	Potassium oxalate	P-273	
	Sodium chloride	S-271	
	Sodium citrate	S-279	
	Sulfanilic acid	A-296	
	L-Tyrosine	T-369	

*Address: Cockeysville, Maryland. Another manufacturer of similar products is Difco Laboratories, Detroit, Michigan.

†Address: St. Louis, Missouri.

4. Cost of Bacteriological Examination

In setting up a laboratory it should be decided whether media are to be made on the premises or purchased from a supply house. Most small laboratories find the availability of prepared media an invaluable convenience. Below are presented the approximate costs of presumptive identification of bacteria.

A. Media prepared in laboratory

Materials:

MacConkey agar	$ 9.90/lb	450 plates (20 ml/plate)	$0.02/plate
Trypticase soy agar	$10.00/lb	500 plates (20 ml/plate)	$0.02/plate
TSI agar	$10.00/lb	700 tubes (10 ml/tube)	$0.02/tube
Thioglycolate fluid	$10.00/lb	700 tubes (10 ml/tube)	$0.02/tube
Disposable petri dishes	$20.00/500 plates		$0.04/plate
Disposable tubes	$33.50/1000 tubes		$0.04/tube
Sensitivity discs			$0.03/disc
Sterile swabs	$ 2.00/100 swabs		

Cost of Investigating One Culture:

Isolation onto blood and MacConkey agar	$0.12
Sensitivity study on blood agar	$0.06
Discs (6)	$0.18
TSI tube and agar	$0.06
Thioglycolate tube and broth	$0.06
Swabs	$0.04
Microscope slide	$0.02
	$0.54

B. Prepared media purchased

Materials:

Blood agar plates	$ 8.30/20 plates	$0.42/plate

MacConkey agar plates	$ 7.00/20 plates	$0.35/plate
Divided plates (blood and MacConkey)	$10.50/20 plates	$0.50/plate
TSI tube	$ 2.95/10 tubes	$0.30/tube
Thioglycolate tube	$ 2.95/10 tubes	$0.30/tube

Cost of Investigating One Culture:

Isolation onto blood and MacConkey agar	$0.77
Sensitivity study on blood agar	$0.42
Sensitivity discs (6)	$0.18
TSI tubes	$0.30
Thioglycolate tubes	$0.30
Swabs	$0.04
Microscope slides	$0.02
	$2.13

7

Reagent Preparation, Techniques, and Interpretation of Tests

1. Anaerobic Atmosphere

Reagents and Materials

1. A 1.5-liter, wide-mouthed container with an air-tight lid. (A 3-lb peanut butter jar has proved ideal.)
2. A 100-ml beaker or small container.
3. A small (2 cm diameter) receptacle.
4. 22.5 ml of 15% H_2SO_4. (Add 15 ml of concentrated H_2SO_4 to 85 ml of water.)
5. 2.25 g of finely powdered chromium metal (100 mesh).
6. 0.75 g of sodium carbonate.

Technique

1. Pour sulfuric acid into the small beaker.
2. Add the chromium powder.
3. Place the sodium carbonate in a small receptacle (a 2-cm bottle cap or a small piece of paper is acceptable) and suspend the receptacle in the beaker in such a way that it can easily be tipped into the acid mixture.
4. Place the beaker and its contents in the jar.
5. Lay the inoculated plate or plates on or next to the beaker.
6. Screw the lid of the jar on firmly. (It is advisable to smear the inside rim of the lid with vasoline to obtain a good seal.)
7. After 15–30 min, if the lid is sufficiently air tight, moisture will form on the inside of the beaker and often on the jar. When this moisture

is evident, tip or shake the suspended receptacle of sodium carbonate into the acid chromium mixture.

8. Incubate at 37°C overnight for *Clostridium*; at least two or three days for the gram-negative anaerobes.*

2. Bacitracin Sensitivity Test (Presumptive Identification of Group A *Streptococcus*; *Streptococcus pyogenes*)

Materials

Taxo A discs.

Technique

1. Inoculate beta hemolytic *Streptococcus* onto blood agar or trypticase soy agar plate. Apply Taxo disc A aseptically onto the area of inoculation.
2. Group A *Streptococcus* are inhibited in the presence of low concentration of bacitracin and will, therefore, show zones of no growth around discs.

3. Blood Collection and Storage

Defibrinated blood is frequently recommended, but in our experience it is equally satisfactory and more convenient to draw the blood into a sterile anticoagulant.

Materials

1. Acid citrate dextrose (ACD) solution: Dissolve 13.2 g of sodium citrate, 4.8 g of citric acid, and 14.7 g of dextrose in 1 liter of water.
2. 100-ml (4-oz) bottles

Preparation

1. Into a 100-ml screw-cap bottle, dispense 20 ml of ACD solution.
2. Replace the lid loosely on the bottle and sterilize at 15-lb steam pressure for 15 min.
3. Tighten the lid and permit the anticoagulant to cool.

---

*Another anaerobic system (Gaspac, BBL Division of BioQuest, Cockeysville, Maryland) is available. This system is excellent; where cost is not a consideration, it is to be preferred to the system described above.

Technique

Add 80 ml of aseptically drawn blood to the sterile ACD solution and mix well. Sterile blood should be kept at 4°C and is usable for at least two months.

4. Blood Agar

Preparation

1. Dissolve 40 g of trypticase soy agar in 1 liter of water.
2. Autoclave at 15-lb steam pressure for 15 min.
3. Cool the agar to 45°C or 50°C, ideally by placing it in a 50°C water bath for approximately one hour.
4. Disinfect the bench surface where plates are to be poured by liberally sponging with a 1 : 200 dilution of Roccal or Amphyl.
5. Warm 50 ml of blood to approximately 50°C. Using an aseptic technique, remove several loopfuls of blood and examine microscopically for evidence of bacilli. If sterile, add blood to agar.
6. Mix well and dispense approximately 20 ml into sterile petri dishes. If storage for several weeks is anticipated, 25 ml is advisable, since the effect of drying is minimized when the larger quantity of agar is used.
7. Immediately after the plates are poured (before solidification begins), flame the surface of the agar with a Bunsen burner. The purpose of this is to remove the bubbles from the surface of the agar.
8. When the agar has solidified, invert the plates and incubate at 37°C for 24–48 hr. Discard any plates showing bacterial or fungal growth.
9. To store the plates, invert them, and keep them at 4°C until ready for use.

5. Camp Test

Reagents

1. Known beta hemolytic *Staphylococcus* culture.
2. Blood agar culture plate.

Technique

1. Streak a culture of beta hemolytic *Staphylococcus* in a single wide straight line across the diameter of a blood agar plate.

2. Inoculate the *Streptococcus* to be tested in a single straight line at right angles to the *Staphylococcus* inoculation line. The *Streptococcus* inoculation should come to within one-eighth inch of the *Staphylococcus* inoculation line.
3. As many as 8 or 10 *streptococci* may be tested at one time. Incubate at 37°C for 24 hr.
4. In a positive result the confluence of the hemolytic zones of the *Staphylococcus* and *Streptococcus* merge and form a wide semicircular area of hemolysis. In a negative result the hemolytic zones at the confluence remain discrete.

6. Carbohydrate Fermentation Studies

Preparation of Medium

1. Suspend 28.5 g of cysteine trypticase agar (CTA) medium in 1 liter of distilled water.
2. Bring into solution by heating and dispense in about 5 ml amounts into screw-cap tubes.
3. Autoclave at not more than 12-lb steam pressure for 15 min and allow to cool in an upright position.

Technique

1. Aseptically transfer Taxo discs impregnated with the desired carbohydrate to the medium.
2. Inoculate tubes by stabbing to about one half the depth of the medium. As the inoculating needle goes into the medium, push the disc aside and into the medium somewhat.
3. Reactions are usually evident in 24–48 hr. A loss of the red color, beginning near the disc, is evidence of fermentation of the carbohydrate.

7. Casein Utilization

Preparation of Casein Agar

1. Dissolve 10 g of skim milk powder in 100 ml of distilled water.
2. Suspend 2 g of dehydrated agar in another 100 ml of distilled water.
3. Autoclave the two solutions at 15-lb steam pressure for 15 min.
4. Cool to about 45°–50°C and mix the two solutions.

5. Pour into sterile petri plates.
6. If bubbles appear on the agar surface, flame briefly with the Bunsen burner before the agar begins to solidify.

Technique

1. Inoculate two plates with the gram-positive branching organism. Inoculate aerobically, one plate at room temperature, the other at 37°C.
2. Observe for clearing of the casein.
3. *Streptomyces* spp. characteristically hydrolyze casein in one to three days. *Nocardia brasiliensis* may clear the agar slowly, never in less than four days. *Nocardia asteroides* does not hydrolyze casein.

8. Catalase Test

Technique

1. Add approximately 1 ml of 3% hydrogen peroxide (30% hydrogen peroxide diluted 1 : 10 with distilled water) to good growth on a TSI slant.
2. A definite bubbling reaction is positive.
3. Testing for catalase on blood agar is permissible if a nonhemolytic organism is being used. Keep in mind that a weak positive reaction may be expected from the blood in the agar.

9. Citrate Utilization

Preparation of Citrate Agar

1. Suspend 24.2 g of Simmon citrate agar media in 1 liter of distilled water. Bring into solution by heating.
2. Dispense approximately 5 ml into small screw-cap tubes and autoclave at 15-lb steam pressure for 15 min.
3. Immediately after removing them from the autoclave tilt the tubes to about 45° until agar has solidified, producing a slanted surface.

Technique

1. Inoculate by stabbing the butt and streaking the slant.
2. Only those organisms capable of utilizing citrate as a sole source of carbon will grow on this agar. Appearance of visible growth is

usually accompanied by an alkaline (blue) change of the indicator. Organisms are considered citrate negative if there has been no growth after four days of incubation at 37°C.

10. Coagulase Test

Reagents

1. Rabbit or human plasma. This is most satisfactorily purchased as coagulation control plasma.
2. For economy, this lyophilized plasma can be diluted to at least three times that recommended for coagulation tests by the manufacturer.

Technique

1. Place 0.5 ml of the diluted plasma in a sterile tube.
2. Add a loopful of the organism being tested and mix with the plasma.
3. Incubate at 37°C.
4. Clotting is usually evident in two to three hours for coagulase-positive organisms, but overnight incubation may be necessary when only a small amount of coagulase is present.

11. Decarboxylase Production Test

Preparation of Medium

1. Suspend 3.1 g of decarboxylase broth base in 300 ml of water and dissolve by heating.
2. Divide into two equal portions and add 0.5 g of L-lysine to one portion and 0.5 g of L-ornithine to the other. No pH adjustment is necessary.
3. Dispense in 5-ml amounts into screw-cap tubes and autoclave at 15-lb steam pressure for 15 min.

Technique

1. Introduce a small amount of inoculum into the depth of the tube.
2. Incubate at 37°C.
3. This medium gives valid results only with glucose-fermenting organisms. Acidification of the medium results in a prompt change from the original purple color to yellow. This reaction occurs with all glucose-fermenting organisms regardless of their decarboxylase activity. Those organisms producing decarboxylase are able to re-

alkalinize the medium, restoring the purple color. Therefore, the endpoint is either yellow (negative) or purple (positive). Most decarboxylase-positive organisms produce this definite color change within 24 hr, but a final report of negative should be rendered only after four days of incubation.

12. Dispensing Media

Equipment

1. Pipetting syringe complete with rubber tube.
2. Required quantity of culture plates or tubes.

Technique

1. Set the adjustment on the syringe for the volume to be dispensed.
2. Seal the syringe and rubber tube in paper or cloth wrapping.
3. Autoclave at 15-lb steam pressure for 15 min; cool.
4. Wipe down the bench surface where the medium is to be dispensed with 1 : 200 solution of Roccal or Amphyl and allow to dry.
5. Position the culture plates or tubes on the left-hand side of the work area and remove their protective coverings.
6. Position the agar to be dispensed on the right-hand side of the work area.
7. Break the seal on the syringe wrapping, unwrap the syringe being careful not to let it touch anything, and then gently lower the tube onto the agar. Fill the syringe with medium.
8. Pick up the plate or tube with your left hand, remove the lid, dispense the medium, and immediately replace the lid.
9. When finished dispensing, flush the syringe several times with hot water so that agar will not solidify around the rubber valves.

13. Media for Cultivating *Hemophilus*

Technique

1. *Hemophilus* organisms of veterinary importance grow adequately on sheep and horse blood agar. When the blood from other species is used in preparing blood agar plates, it is essential that X- (hemin) and V- (diphosphopyridine nucleotide) factors are provided for the nutritionally fastidious *Hemophilus* organisms.
2. Commercial strips are available (Taxo strips) in which the X- and V-factors have been impregnated. These provide a simple means of

isolation and/or differentiation of *Hemophilus* organisms. When the organism is placed on the plate, preferably on agar without blood, the desired factor is diffused into the agar and the organisms growth requirements may be observed.

14. Indole Production

Reagent

Ehrlich reagent: Dissolve 4 g of *p*-dimethylaminobenzaldehyde in 380 ml of 95% ethyl alcohol. Cautiously add 80 ml of concentrated HCl.

Preparation

1. Dissolve 36 g of SIM (sulfide indole motility) medium in 1 liter of distilled water by heating.
2. Dispense 5–10 ml into tubes.
3. Sterilize at 15-lb steam pressure (121°C) for 15 min.
4. Allow the tubed medium to solidify in a vertical position.

Technique

1. Inoculate by stabbing with a straight wire to about one-half the depth of the agar. Incubate at 37°C.
2. Overlay a 48-hr growth of the organism on SIM with Ehrlich reagent. Development of a pink to red color is positive for indole.

15. Media for Cultivating *Leptospira*

Fletcher medium base and Stuart broth base are useful in diagnostic studies of *Leptospira*. The dehydrated materials may be purchased together with the *Leptospira* enrichment additive. Since these are not common media, directions may be obtained when the media are purchased. Purchase of prepared media is recommended because it takes a considerable amount of experience to cultivate these organisms.

16. MacConkey Agar Medium

Preparation

1. Suspend 50 g of the dehydrated MacConkey agar in 1 liter of distilled water.

2. Heat to bring into solution and sterilize by autoclaving at 15-lb steam pressure for 15 min.
3. Cool to 45°–50°C and pour into petri plates. The reason for cooling to this temperature is to prevent excessive condensation on the lid of the petri plate. Twenty milliliters per plate is usually satisfactory unless the plates are to be stored for a considerable period of time, in which case more agar should be used per plate.
4. Allow the medium to solidify with the lid partially removed to obtain a dry surface for inoculation if the medium is to be used soon after preparation.
5. To store the plates, invert them and keep them at 4°C until ready for use.

17. Malonate Utilization

Preparation

1. Dissolve 9.3 g of dehydrated malonate broth in 1 liter of distilled water.
2. Dispense in about 5-ml amounts in screw-cap test tubes.
3. Sterilize at 15-lb steam pressure for 15 min.

Technique

1. Inoculate well down into the broth medium and incubate for 48 hr at 37°C.
2. Organisms able to utilize the malonate of this synthetic medium as an energy source produce an alkaline reaction during growth and change the color of the medium from the original green to blue.

18. Microaerophilic Atmosphere

Materials

1. Wide-mouthed jar with a tightly fitting lid. (A 3-lb peanut butter jar is suitable.)
2. Short, thick candle standing upright in a small container.

Preparation

1. Place the inoculated plates in the wide-mouthed jar.
2. Place the candle on top of the plates.

3. Smear the inner side rim of the lid with vasoline to obtain a good seal.
4. Light the candle and fit the lid firmly on the jar.
5. When the candle is extinguished, swirl the jar gently to evenly distribute CO_2 (the carbon dioxide concentration will be approximately 2–3%).
6. Incubate at 37°C.

19. Motility Test

Using Semisolid Media

1. Motility may be determined on any of the following media:
   a. SIM medium employed for the indole test,
   b. nitrate agar employed for the nitrate test,
   c. CTA medium employed for carbohydrate fermentation studies.
2. Inoculate to approximately one-half the depth of the medium, using a straight wire. Incubate at 37°C until good growth occurs.
3. Motility is evidenced by a diffusion of growth from the line of inoculation.

Using Broth Cultures

1. Motility may also be determined by the wet mount method from broth cultures.
2. Inoculate the organism into a tube of trypticase soy broth.
3. Incubate overnight at 37°C.
4. Place one drop of broth growth on a clean microscope slide. Cover with a clean cover slip.
5. Examine microscopically for distinctly motile organisms using high power magnification. (Brownian movement is to be ignored).

20. Media for Cultivating *Mycobacterium*

Materials

Lowenstein-Jenson medium and Petragnani medium, as well as several other media, are in common use for isolating *Mycobacterium*. Such media are best purchased commercially.

Technique

1. Inoculate two tubes by deep stabbing and by streaking the slant.
2. Incubate one tube at room temperature and the other at 37°C.

3. Saprophytic *mycobacterium* grows within three days at 37°C and at room temperature and gives a strong catalase reaction. *Mycobacterium avium* also grows at 37°C and room temperature, usually appearing after from one to two weeks and gives a weak catalase reaction. *Mycobacterium tuberculosis* and *Mycobacterium bovis* grow only at 37°C. The latter two species may be differentiated by animal inoculation. *Mycobacterium tuberculosis* injected subcutaneously into guinea pigs gives rise to a fatal disease. Rabbits and mice are less affected. *Mycobacterium bovis* is virulent for rabbits, mice, and guinea pigs. Differentiation of the less frequently isolated *mycobacteria* depends on their ability or inability to produce chromogens.

21. Media for Cultivating *Mycoplasma*

1. *Mycoplasma* agar base and some selective and nonselective nutrient enrichments may be purchased. Nutritive supplements should include 10% serum and 10% yeast extract. Bacterial inhibitors are essential.
2. Primary isolation is best made in a moist microaerophilic atmosphere and incubation should continue for 21 days before the culture is declared negative. A candle jar containing a saturated paper towel is ideal for keeping the incubation vessel moist.
3. Growth is recognized as "poached-egg" colony formation. A simple way to examine for growth is by placing the agar plate upside down on the microscope stage and viewing the agar surface with a low-power objective.

22. NaCl Broth (6.5%)

Preparation

1. Suspend 30 g of trypticase soy broth powder in 1 liter of distilled water.
2. Add 60 g of sodium chloride (NaCl) and dissolve. This brings the total sodium chloride content to 6.5%.
3. Dispense into screw-cap tubes, approximately 5 ml per tube.
4. Sterilize at 15-lb steam pressure for 15 min.

Technique

1. Inoculate with a gram-positive coccus suspected of being an enterococcus and incubate at 37°C.

2. Growth, evidenced by cloudiness of the inoculated broth in comparison to an uninoculated tube, indicates that the organism is an enterococcus.
3. If no growth is apparent within 48 hr, the organism is not of an enterococcus.

23. Nitrate Reduction Test

Reagents

1. Prepare 200 ml of 5 N acetic acid by adding 56.8 ml of glacial acetic acid to 143 ml of water. Divide into two portions of 100 ml each.
2. Add 0.8 g of sulfanilic acid to 100 ml of 5 N acetic acid.
3. Add 0.5 g of 1-naphthylamine to 100 ml of 5 N acetic acid.

Preparation

1. Add 2 g of agar to 25 g of indole nitrate medium and dissolve in 1 liter of distilled water by heating.
2. Dispense approximately 5 ml into screw-cap tubes.
3. Sterilize at 15-lb steam pressure for 15 min. Allow tubes to cool in a vertical position.

Technique

1. Inoculate by stabbing to approximately one-half the depth of the medium.
2. Test for the presence of nitrite when good growth occurs; usually overnight incubation is sufficient. To test for nitrites, (1) add several drops of reagent 2 above or, (2) add several drops of reagent 3 above.
3. A red color is positive for nitrites.
4. A few bacteria, such as *Pseudomonas* and *Bacillus* species, may actually denitrify nitrate; that is, they may reduce nitrate to nitrite to gaseous nitrogen. Cultures should, therefore, be observed early and frequently.
5. When excessive gas is present, denitrification should be suspected in those cultures giving a negative nitrite test. Zinc dust should then be added to these cultures. If the reaction is still negative after the addition of zinc dust, nitrates have been previously reduced to gaseous nitrogen by the organism and the organism is called nitrate

positive. If after the addition of the zinc dust a red color develops, the organism is nitrate negative.

24. Oxidation-Fermentation (OF) Reaction

Preparation of Medium

1. Suspend 9.6 g of OF basal medium in 1 liter of distilled water.
2. Add 10 g of dextrose and bring into solution by heating.
3. Dispense 5-ml amounts into screw-cap tubes.
4. Sterilize at 12-lb steam pressure (118°C) for 15 min.

Technique

1. Inoculate two tubes with the organism in question, stabbing well down into the medium.
2. Overlay the medium in one tube with approximately 0.5 ml of sterile paraffin oil.
3. Incubate both tubes at 37°C.
4. Observe after from 12 to 48 hr for acidification (a change from the original blue to yellow).
5. Organisms utilizing glucose fermentatively produce acidification in the covered tube as well as in the open one; the reaction is recorded as F.
6. Those organisms whose utilization of glucose is oxidative are able to utilize only the carbohydrate in the open tube; the reaction is recorded as O.
7. When growth is evident in the medium but no color change has occurred, the organism lacks the ability to utilize glucose.

25. Oxidase Production

Preparation

1. A fresh 0.5% solution of tetramethylparaphenylene diamine dihydrochloride is the more sensitive of the several reagents available.
2. A 0.5% aqueous solution of *p*-aminodimethylanaline oxalate is fairly sensitive and is comparatively stable. The solution, after preparation, is allowed to stand at room temperature until a pink color develops. It is then stored in the refrigerator. It will give satisfactory results for several weeks.
3. Commercial supply houses such as BBL, Difco, and Warner-Chil-

cott offer prepared discs and strips for the oxidase test. These are convenient, and their use is advised for the small clinical practice. Not all of these are as sensitive as the liquid reagents, however, and in the case of *Pasteurella multocida*, a common veterinary pathogen, may give a negative reaction.

Technique

1. Apply a few drops of liquid reagent directly to growth on the blood agar plate or smear a few colonies on a paper towel and apply the reagent.
2. Colonies producing cytochrome oxidase become pink and turn to red and sometimes black within a few minutes.
3. The discs and strips give an evident rose or purplish color when smeared with an organism producing oxidase. The discs may also be moistened and placed on the blood agar plate near the colony being studied. A period of incubation at 37°C is recommended when the latter approach is used, as room temperature delays the reaction.

26. Media for Cultivating *Pasteurella tularensis*

Preparation

1. Dissolve 51 g of cystine heart agar in 1 liter of distilled water by heating.
2. Sterilize at 15-lb steam pressure for 15 min.
3. Cool the agar to 80°C.
4. Add approximately 50 ml of blood.
5. Maintain the 80°C temperature for approximately 10 min to form chocolate agar.
6. Cool to 45°–50°C and pour into plates using 20–25 ml per plate.

27. Phenylethyl Alcohol Agar (PEA) Medium

Preparation

1. Dissolve 42.5 g of phenylethyl alcohol agar in 1 liter of distilled water.
2. Sterilize at 12–15-lb steam pressure for 15 min.
3. Disinfect the bench surface where plates are to be poured by liberally sponging with 1 : 100 dilution of Roccal or Amphyl.

4. Cool to 45°–50°C and add 50 ml of blood.
5. Mix well and dispense into sterile petri plates with approximately 20 ml per plate.
6. Immediately after the plates are poured, flame the surface briefly with a Bunsen burner to remove bubbles.
7. When the agar has solidified, invert the plates and incubate at 37°C for 24–48 hr. Discard any plates showing bacterial or fungal growth.
8. For storage, invert the plates and keep them at 4°C until ready for use.
9. This medium is designed for isolation of gram-positive organisms with inhibition of gram negatives. It is especially useful for recovery of gram-positive organisms which have been overgrown by *Proteus*.

28. Phytone Medium

Preparation

1. Place approximately 1 g of cooked meal phytone medium in a dry screw-capped tube.
2. Add approximately 10 ml of water.
3. Rotate the tubes and allow them to stand for about 15 min. The medium forms a suspension.
4. Add a thin layer, approximately one-fourth of an inch, of sealing material (such as paraffin oil; Vaspar, a mixture of equal parts of vaseline and paraffin; etc.).
5. Sterilize at 15-lb steam pressure for 15 min.
6. This medium is used for (a) encouraging spore formation, (b) establishing proteolysis, (c) establishing sulfide production.

29. Test for Proteolysis

Materials

Tubes of phytone medium.

Technique

1. Inoculate approximately 0.1 ml of the thioglycolate broth growth of the organism to be tested, using a sterile pipette, and incubate for 24 hr.
2. Proteolysis is evidenced by digestion of meat particles.

30. Optochin Sensitivity Test (Presumptive Identification of *Pneumococci*)

Materials

Taxo P discs.

Technique

1. Inoculate alpha hemolytic cocci onto a blood agar or trypticase soy agar plate. Apply a Taxo P disc aseptically to the area of inoculation.
2. Pneumococci are inhibited in the presence of ethylhydrocupreine hydrochloride (optochin) and will, therefore, show a zone of no growth around the Taxo P disc.

31. *Streptococcus faecalis* (SF) Broth

Preparation

1. Dissolve 36 g of SF medium in 1 liter of distilled water.
2. Dispense into screw-cap test tubes in approximately 5-ml amounts.
3. Autoclave at 15-lb steam pressure for 15 min.

Technique

1. Inoculate gram-positive cocci, suspected of being enterococci, well down into the medium.
2. Incubate at 37°C for at least 48 hr unless an acid change, evidenced by a change from the original bromcresol purple to yellow, occurs earlier. Those organisms growing in, and acidifying, the medium are considered enterococci.

32. *Salmonella* Agglutination Test

Reagents

Salmonella O antisera, polyvalent A-I.

Technique

1. Put a few drops of saline in the TSI tube of suspected *Salmonella.* Shake gently until the saline turns cloudy with the organism.
2. Place two drops of the saline suspension of organism on a clean glass slide. One drop is for the test; the other is for the control.

3. To the test saline (bacterial mixture) add a small drop of *Salmonella* antiserum. Mix.
4. Tilt the slide carefully back and forth observing both the test and control suspensions for agglutination. If agglutination appears within several minutes in the test suspension but not in the control, the test is positive.

33. Selenite Broth

Preparation

1. Sterilize large (15–20 ml) screw-cap tubes at 15-lb steam pressure.
2. Suspend 23 g of selenite cystine broth or selenite-F broth in 1 liter of distilled water and heat to dissolve completely.
3. Dispense into sterile tubes, 10 ml per tube. Do not autoclave.
4. The tubed medium may be used as soon as it cools. If the medium is to be stored, heat it in flowing steam for 15 min before storage. Store at 4°C with lids fastened tightly.

Technique

1. Add 1–2 g of the specimen to a tube of selenite broth and incubate at 37°C for 12–24 hr.
2. Inoculate a MacConkey agar plate from the broth culture, making the transfer with a sterile cotton-tipped applicator stick. Streak for isolated colonies with a wire loop.
3. Incubate the MacConkey plate overnight at 37°C. Identification of *Salmonella* is made as shown in Table 1.

34. Spore Formation

Materials

Tubes of phytone medium.

Technique

1. Inoculate approximately 0.1 ml of the thioglycolate broth growth of the organism to be tested, using a sterile pipette, and incubate for 24 hr.
2. Spore formation readily occurs in this medium.
3. Stain as in the following section.

35. Spore Stain

Reagents

1. Ziehl–Neelsen carbol fuchsin
   A. Dissolve 0.3 g of basic fuchsin in 10 ml of 95% ethyl alcohol.
   B. Dissolve 4.5 g of phenol in 90 ml of water.
   Mix A and B. Let stand for 24 hr and filter. The solution remains stable indefinitely.
2. 30% ferric chloride
   Dissolve 30 g of ferric chloride in 100 ml of water.
3. 5% sodium sulfite
   Dissolve 5 g of sodium sulfite in 100 ml of water.
4. 1% methylene blue
   Dissolve 1 g of methylene blue in 100 ml of water.

Technique

1. Place a drop of phytone medium growth of organism on a clean glass slide. Air dry.
2. Heat fix carefully with a minimum amount of heat.
3. Stain with Ziehl–Neelsen carbol fuchsin for 3 min, heating gently until slight steaming is observed.
4. Wash in water.
5. Treat with ferric chloride solution for 1 min.
6. Treat with sodium sulfite solution for 30 sec.
7. Wash in water.
8. Counterstain with methylene blue solution for 1 min.
9. Wash in water.
10. Blot or air dry and examine with oil immersion objective.
11. Spores retain the red color of the carbol fuchsin. The protoplasm of the bacteria stains with the blue of the counterstain.

36. Sulfide Production of *Clostridium* sp.

Materials

Tubes of phytone medium.

Technique

1. Inoculate approximately 0.1 ml of the thioglycolate broth growth of the organism to be tested, using a sterile pipette, and incubate for 24 hr.
2. Sulfide production is shown by blackening of the medium.

37. Tetrathionate Broth

Reagents

Iodine solution: iodine, 6 g; potassium iodide, 5 g; water, 20 ml.

Preparation

1. Suspend 46 g of tetrathionate broth base in 1 liter of distilled water. Mix thoroughly.
2. Heat to boiling.
3. Cool to a temperature of less than 45°C.
4. Dispense in either 10-ml amounts in screw-cap tubes or 100-ml amounts in a 250-ml flask with a screw-cap.
5. Prior to use, add 2–4 drops of iodine solution to 10 ml of broth and mix well, or add 2 ml to 100 ml of broth. Once iodine is added, the medium must be used on the day of preparation.

Technique for Salmonella *Isolation*

1. Into 10-ml broth introduce a rectal swab or 1 or 2 g of feces and swirl for few minutes. Remove the swab. Incubate at 37°C.
2. If using 100-ml broth, add 30 g of feces. Incubate at 37°C.
3. After 6 to 24 hr of incubation, subculture onto MacConkey agar.

38. Thioglycolate Broth

Preparation

1. Dissolve 24 g of thioglycolate medium in 1 liter of distilled water.
2. Dispense in 10–15-ml amounts in screw-cap tubes.
3. Sterilize at 15-lb steam pressure for 15 min.

39. Triple Sugar Iron (TSI) Agar

Preparation

1. Suspend 60 g of TSI medium in 1 liter of distilled water.
2. Bring into solution by heating, and dispense approximately 5 ml into screw-cap tubes.
3. Sterilize at not more than 12-lb steam pressure for 15 min.
4. Allow the agar to solidify with the tubes held at a 45° angle so that a slanted surface and a deep butt is formed.

Technique

1. Using a straight wire, inoculate by stabbing the butt and streaking the slant. Incubate at 37°C.
2. Fermentative utilization of glucose is evidenced by yellowing of the butt.
3. H_2S production is shown as blackening of the medium. These reactions are usually apparent after 24 hr of incubation.

40. Trypticase Soy Agar Medium

Preparation

1. Dissolve 40 g of trypticase soy agar in 1 liter of water.
2. Autoclave at 15-lb steam pressure for 15 min.
3. Cool the agar to 45°–50°C, ideally by placing it in a 50°C water bath for approximately 1 hr.
4. Disinfect the bench surface where the plates are to be poured by liberally sponging with a 1 : 200 dilution of Roccal or Amphyl.
5. Mix well and dispense approximately 20 ml into sterile petri dishes. If storage for several weeks is anticipated, 25 ml is advisable as the effect of drying is minimized when the larger quantity of agar is used.
6. Immediately after the plates are poured (before solidification begins), flame the surface of the agar with a Bunsen burner. This removes the bubbles from the surface of the agar.
7. When the agar has solidified, invert the plates and incubate at 37°C for 24–48 hr. Discard any plates showing bacterial or fungal growth.
8. To store them, invert the plates and keep them at 4°C until ready for use.

41. Trypticase Soy Broth

Preparation

1. Dissolve 27.5 g of trypticase soy broth base in 1 liter of distilled water.
2. Dispense in 2–3-ml amounts in small screw-cap tubes.
3. Sterilize at 15-lb steam pressure for 15 min.

42. Tyrosine Utilization

Preparation of Medium

1. To 100 ml of distilled water, add 4 g of trypticase soy agar and 0.5 g of L-tyrosine.
2. Sterilize at 15-lb steam pressure for 15 min.
3. Cool to 45°–50°C.
4. Pour into sterile petri plates, agitating the flask gently to maintain an even distribution of the insoluble tyrosine.
5. If the surface of the freshly poured agar has bubbles, flame briefly with a Bunsen burner before solidification of the agar has begun.

Technique

1. Inoculate two plates with the gram-positive branching organism. Incubate aerobically, one plate at room temperature and the other at 37°C.
2. Observe for disappearance of the tyrosine crystals underneath and around colonies after 14 and 21 days of incubation.
3. *Nocardia* sp. rarely decompose tyrosine, whereas *Streptomyces* seldom fail to do so.

43. Urease Production

Preparation of Urea Agar

1. Dissolve 29 g of urea agar base in 100 ml of distilled water.
2. Filter sterilize.
3. Dissolve 15 g of agar in 900 ml of distilled water.
4. Autoclave at 15-lb steam pressure for 15 min.
5. Cool to about 50°C.
6. Aseptically add the 100-ml urea agar base from step 1 and mix thoroughly. At pH of 6.8 to 7.0, the medium should have a light pinkish-yellow color. If the color is a definite pink, add a small amount of HCl to bring it to the pinkish-yellow color.
7. Dispense aseptically into small sterile screw-cap tubes.
8. Allow the tubed medium to cool, holding the tubes at a 45° angle so that the surface of the agar is slanted.
9. Store urea agar slants in a refrigerator until used.

Technique

1. Inoculate heavily over the surface of the slant without stabbing into the butt. The butt serves as the negative control. Incubate at 37°C.
2. Organisms capable of splitting urea release ammonia and therefore alkalinize and cause a red color change in the slant of the agar. *Proteus* typically produces a positive reaction in from 2 to 4 hr. The reaction of enteric organisms should be observed after overnight incubation; but with such organisms as *Brucella*, several days' incubation may be necessary.

44. Voges–Proskauer Reaction

Preparation of MR–VP Broth

1. Dissolve 17 g of MR–VP broth powder in 1 liter of distilled water.
2. Dispense into small screw-cap tubes, approximately 5 ml per tube.
3. Sterilize at not more than 15-lb steam pressure for 15 min.

Reagents

1. Dissolve 5 g of 1-naphthol in 100 ml of absolute ethyl alcohol.
2. Dissolve 40 g of potassium hydroxide in 100 ml of water. Add 0.3 g of creatine, and mix. (This is a very caustic solution.)

Procedure

1. Inoculate a tube of MR–VP broth with the organism being tested, and incubate for 48 hr at 37°C.
2. Add 0.6 ml of a solution of 5% 1-naphthol in absolute ethyl alcohol and 0.2 ml of a solution of 0.3% creatine in 40% KOH.
3. A bright orange, reddish color developing in 5–10 min is positive, denoting the formation of acetylmethylcarbinol by the organism.

8

Evaluation of Effectiveness of Chemotherapeutic Agents

1. Sensitivity Testing

The susceptibility of an organism to chemotherapeutic agents is usually determined by the disc method. Paper discs impregnated with known amounts of chemotherapeutic agents are placed on a culture medium that has been uniformly inoculated with the bacteria being tested. During incubation the agent diffuses into the agar producing a concentration gradient. If the agent prevents the development of the organism, a clear zone of inhibition around the disc is observed. A number of discs are applied simultaneously to different portions of the culture plate to survey the spectrum of agents to which the test organism is sensitive. Ideally, the amounts of agent on the paper disc should correspond to the blood level of the agent which is usually achieved with conventional dosage. Organisms are reported as either sensitive or resistant.

Most veterinary bacteriology laboratories routinely perform sensitivity testing. However, some clinical pathologists feel that the results are meaningless. Criticisms that have been made against the procedure are:

1. causative organisms may not be present in sufficient numbers in a mixed culture to give reliable results;
2. the original specimen may not in fact yield a primary pathogen;
3. diffusion of chemotherapeutic agents into the agar is not uniform;
4. results from different laboratories often are not comparable.

The criticism that the pathogen may not be present in sufficient numbers is academic. In many clinical situations there is an urgent need to begin appropriate antibiotic therapy, in which case the sensitivity test is performed on the original specimen even if it is a mixed culture. The composition of a mixed bacterial population at the site of infection is unknown. The primary pathogen may be present there in small numbers. Therefore a chemotherapeutic agent that will prevent growth of all organisms in a mixed culture should be used. It is preferable to study pure cultures of bacterial isolates from clinical material. When the individual bacterial species from a mixed culture have been isolated and identified, they should be restudied separately for sensitivity determinations.

The criticisms concerning the diffusion of antibiotics as a cause of variable results have as a basis the suggestion that the width of the zone of inhibition is due to many uncontrolled factors. Primarily three factors influence the width of the zone of inhibition: the amount of chemotherapeutic agent impregnated on the paper disc, the density of colony growth on the surface of the agar, and the diffusion of the drug through the agar. The most important factor affecting reproducibility of the sensitivity test is the quantity of drug on the paper disc. Recent evidence from a nationwide survey shows that a high degree of reproducibility and reliability can be achieved with standardized impregnated discs. Factors such as composition of the agar medium, storage, volume of agar poured onto the culture plate, and concentration of blood in the agar have no appreciable influence on the size of the zone of inhibition. The bacteriologist must standardize the density of the colony growth used in the sensitivity test. Although it has no effect on the immediate clinical interpretation whether confluent colonies or heavy dense growth was used, it is essential that standardization of colony density be achieved so that any change in the in vitro effectiveness of an agent can be recognized.

With the proliferation of drugs available to the clinician, it is often difficult to decide which agents should be tested and what concentration of those agents on the chemotherapeutically impregnated discs should be used. The standard dispenser for the 10-cm culture plate delivers eight discs. Since most veterinary practices have less than eight drugs in common use, one drug susceptibility test is adequate. In mixed practices it may be more convenient to have one dispenser loaded with discs of drugs used in small animal therapy and another loaded with those used in farm animal practice. The high-concentration antibiotic discs should be used.

Strains resistant to antibiotics in present use are now becoming increasingly common; antibiotic resistant *Pseudomonas*, *Staphylococcus*, and *Salmonella*, for example, are now common. It is now an avowed principle in veterinary clinical medicine that antibiotics should be used as little as possible; and when they are used, they should be given in large doses and their use stopped as soon as possible. For this reason, clinicians should use only those drugs that have clear-cut zones of inhibition. Comparison of the width of zone of inhibition of different drugs as a measure of in vivo efficacy is valueless. The width of the zone of inhibition provides an evaluation of the relative sensitivity of an organism to a drug. Thus a decrease in the width of the zone of inhibition under standard sensitivity testing conditions suggests a changing susceptibility to a therapeutic agent. Since the veterinarian has a responsibility to both his patient and his client to offer the most efficient therapy, he should be aware of any change in sensitivity results.

It is sometimes thought that in vitro testing does not indicate in vivo efficacy. When such a possibility is being considered, the clinician must be certain that the specimen sent to the laboratory is representative of the bacterial problem.

2. Materials for Sensitivity Testing

1. Agar plate: trypticase soy agar, MacConkey agar, or PEA
2. Tube of trypticase soy broth
3. Sterile cotton-tipped applicator stick
4. Antibiotic discs*
5. Antibiotic disc dispenser*

3. Technique for Sensitivity Testing

1. Transfer a colony of the organism to be tested into a tube of sterile trypticase soy broth. Mix well.† If the sensitivity test is to be performed on the original specimen, dip the specimen directly into the broth.
2. Dip a sterile cotton-tipped applicator stick into the broth suspension and streak the surface of an agar plate evenly. Trypticase soy agar plates are usually used, but MacConkey agar plates or PEA plates may be preferred when selective growth will be an advantage.
3. Using aseptic precautions, place the antibiotic discs on the agar and gently press each disc onto the agar surface. Discs should be spaced

*These are manufactured by BBL, Division of Bioquest, Cockeysville, Maryland, and are sold by most supply houses.

†For those organisms having very small colonies, such as *Streptococcus*, incubate the inoculated broth at 37°C for approximately 4–6 hr to provide a sufficiently heavy inoculum.

farther apart for the more slowly growing organisms, since their inhibition zones tend to be larger.

4. Incubate until growth occurs and examine for clear zones around the discs—evidence of inhibition of growth by the antibiotic.
5. Sensitivity readings often are hastened by swabbing an agar plate heavily with the contaminated material and placing the discs on the inoculated areas. Particularly with slowly growing organisms, this may be the preferred method, since the delay caused by prior isolation may make the final sensitivity readings and report of little or no value to the clinician.

9

Illustrative Cases

Case 1

Species: Canine, adult female

History/Diagnosis

1. Blastomycosis
2. Pericarditis

Specimens

1. Material from abscess in chest
2. Pleural fluid

Laboratory Findings

1. The exudate contained small firm yellow particles, sulfur granules, among the cellular debris. Direct smear of sulfur granules showed branching gram-positive filaments. These did not retain the original stain with the acid-fast method.
2. Culture plates were examined after 72 hr of incubation in aerobic and anaerobic atmospheres.
3. No growth was obtained on MacConkey agar.
4. Blood agar cultures from the abscess showed moderate growth of very small white colonies which appeared to be sunk into the agar. No hemolysis. Anaerobiosis hindered growth; very light colony growth was observed. Cultures from pleural fluid were negative.
5. Morphology and gram stain indicated *Nocardia* spp. Because the organism was isolated from the sulfur granules, its characteristic morphology, aerobic growth, and stain indicated *Nocardia* spp.
6. This case is of interest because *Nocardia* is most frequently isolated from cattle.
7. No sensitivity studies were done.

Organism: *Nocardia*

Case 2

Species: Equine adult female

History/Diagnosis: Infertility

Specimen: Cervical swab

Laboratory Findings

1. MacConkey agar cultures showed heavy growth of small colorless colonies, estimated less than 1 mm in diameter.
2. Blood agar cultures showed heavy growth of grayish white, nonhemolytic colonies in pure culture.
3. Organism was diplococcoid and stained gram negative.
4. TSI agar was inoculated. No change had occurred after 48 hr of incubation.
5. Urea agar was inoculated. No urease was produced.
6. MacConkey agar was inoculated. Small colorless or transparent colonies with a faint purplish tint appeared at first to be lactose fermenters. This second culture was made to confirm that no lactase fermentation was previously observed.
7. Trypticase soy broth was inoculated. The organism was nonmotile.
8. The oxidase test was negative.
9. No reaction occurred on OF medium.
10. The test for nitrate reduction was negative.

Organism: *Mima polymorpha*

Sensitivity

Furaltadone: R*
Neomycin: S*
Penicillin: R
Streptomycin: S
Sulfathiazole: R
Terramycin: S
Tetracycline: S

Case 3

Species: Equine, adult female

*R = resistant, S = sensitive.

History/Diagnosis: Infertility

Specimen: Cervical swab

Laboratory Findings

1. After 24 hr of incubation, heavy growth of small, grayish-white non-hemolytic colonies was seen on blood agar. No colony growth was observed on MacConkey agar.
2. Smear preparation showed as gram-negative, pleomorphic coccobacilli.
3. No change in the butt of TSI agar slant was observed 24 hr after subculture. This suggested that the organism was in the *Brucella, Moraxella, Mima, Actinobacillus* group.
4. A subculture from the blood agar plate was made to MacConkey agar. After 24 hr no growth was visible. After 48 hr a few, non-lactose-fermenting colonies were seen.
5. The organism was found to have the following characteristics:
   (a) nitrate reduction: negative,
   (b) urease production: positive,
   (c) oxidase production: positive,
   (d) nonutilization of OF medium,
   (e) no motility.
6. The organism was suspected to be *Mima* because of its morphology. Other more detailed studies were made to establish a profile of its characteristics. A reference laboratory also confirmed it to be *Mima.*
7. This is an interesting isolate, because urease production is so rare that it is shown as negative in Table 1. Another feature of the isolate was oxidase production.

Organism: *Mima polymorpha* var. *oxidans*

Sensitivity

Furaltadone, S
Neomycin, S
Penicillin, S
Streptomycin, R
Sulfathiazole, R
Terramycin, R
Tetracycline, S

Case 4

Species: Bear, one-year-old male

History/Diagnosis: Infection of surgical wound

Specimen: Material from subcutaneous puncture

Laboratory Findings

1. On MacConkey agar heavy growth of colorless, round, non-lactose-fermenting colonies was seen. The colonies were 1–3 mm in diameter.
2. On blood agar heavy growth of similar, nonhemolytic colonies was seen. Because of the odor, *Proteus* was suspected.
3. Gram-negative rods.
4. When inoculated onto TSI agar, H_2S was produced.
5. When inoculated onto urea agar, there was a rapid urease reaction.

Organism: *Proteus*

Sensitivity

Furaltadone, R
Neomycin, S
Penicillin, S
Streptomycin, S
Sulfathiazole, indefinite
Terramycin, R
Tetracycline, R

Case 5

Species: Canine, female pup (one week old)

History/Diagnosis: Crying constantly; purulent discharge from right eye

Specimen: Swab of purulent discharge

Laboratory Findings

1. After 24 hr of incubation no growth was observed on MacConkey agar.
2. Heavy growth of medium-sized white nonhemolytic colonies in pure culture was seen on blood agar.
3. Gram-positive cocci.

4. Positive catalase and coagulase reactions confirmed the organism as *Staphylococcus aureus*.

Organism: *Staphylococcus aureus*

Sensitivity

Aureomycin, S
Chloramycetin, S
Furadantin, S
Kanamycin, S
Neomycin, S
Penicillin, S
Polymyxin B, R
Terramycin, S

Case 6

Species: Canine, adult female

History/Diagnosis: Chronic otitis externa, seborrhea

Specimen: Swab from external ear canal

Laboratory Findings

1. After 24 hr of incubation the blood agar plate was overrun by a spreading organism, immediately suggestive of *Proteus* sp. A faint greenish pigment was seen in the area of heaviest inoculation. The odor from the plate was not that characteristic of either *Proteus* or *Pseudomonas*.
2. On MacConkey agar there was a heavy growth of colorless non-lactose-fermenting colonies which were well over 1 mm in diameter.
3. At this stage the evidence pointed strongly to a pure culture of *Proteus* but the absence of the *Proteus* odor aroused suspicions. Five TSI agar slants were inoculated from separate colonies from MacConkey agar. All showed no H_2S production and no change in butt. Absence of H_2S production without fermentation of glucose showed that the organism was not *Proteus*.
4. Subculturing from TSI onto blood agar gave pure growth of discrete colonies, green pigment, and, the "fruity" odor of *Pseudomonas*. The oxidase test was positive. OF glucose utilization test was oxidative.
5. This specimen was of interest because examination after 24 hr sug-

gested a pure culture of *Proteus*. The value of MacConkey agar in preventing a swarming growth of *Proteus* was well illustrated. When swarming was inhibited, five colonies picked at random proved to be *Pseudomonas*. Although both organisms are pathogenic in this condition, *Pseudomonas* was dominant in the lesion.

Organism: *Pseudomonas; Proteus*

Sensitivity

Ampicillin, R
Aureomycin, R
Chloromycetin, R
Furadantin, R
Kanamycin, R
Neomycin, S
Penicillin, R
Polymyxin B, S
Terramycin, R

Case 7

Species: Canine, adult female

History/Diagnosis: Pyometra

Specimen: Material aspirated from uterus

Laboratory Findings

1. After 24 hr of incubation heavy growth of red colonies over 1 mm in diameter was seen on MacConkey agar.
2. On blood agar, heavy growth of large grayish-white colonies showing narrow zones of beta hemolysis was seen.
3. Gram-negative rods.
4. Subculture into TSI agar showed the absence of H_2S production and yellow butt.
5. Twenty-four hours after subculture into SIM medium, positive indole reaction was obtained. Proof of indole production is adequate confirmation for *Escherichia coli*.
6. In addition to the minimum tests, the organism showed the following reactions:
   (a) Voges-Proskauer: negative
   (b) citrate: negative

(c) urease: negative
(d) motility: positive

Organism: *Escherichia*

Sensitivity

Ampicillin, S
Aureomycin, S
Chloromycetin, S
Furadantin, S
Kanamycin, S
Neomycin, S
Penicillin, —
Polymyxin B, S
Terromycin, S

Case 8

Species: Bovine, adult male

History/Diagnosis: Pink eye

Specimen: Conjunctival swab

Laboratory Findings

1. No growth was observed after 24 and 48 hr of incubation on MacConkey agar.
2. On blood agar heavy growth of small whitish colonies showing narrow zones of beta hemolysis was seen.
3. Gram stain showed gram-negative coccobacilli with a strong tendency to occur in pairs, but not the coffee-bean arrangement of the *Neisseria* group.
4. The following tests confirmed *Moraxella:*
   (a) no change on TSI agar,
   (b) oxidase production: positive,
   (c) urease: negative,
   (d) no motility,
   (e) nitrate reduction: positive,
   (f) indole: negative.

Organism: *Moraxella bovis*

Sensitivity

Furaltadone, —
Neomycin, —
Penicillin, —
Streptomycin, —
Sulfathiazole, —
Sulfamethizole, —
Terramycin, S
Tetracycline, S

Case 9

Species: Bovine, adult female

History/Diagnosis: Mastitis

Specimen: Milk

Laboratory Findings

1. Microscopic examination of wet smears showed many medium-sized rods, with no motility evident.
2. After 24 hr of incubation, MacConkey agar showed heavy growth of pink, moist, runny colonies, all over 1 mm in diameter. The specimen had a yeasty smell.
3. On blood agar there was a heavy growth of nonhemolytic colonies with no pigmentation.
4. Gram-negative rods.
5. On TSI agar a yellow butt and no H_2S production was seen.
6. *Escherichia*, *Enterobacter*, and *Klebsiella* were considered the most likely possibilities.
7. The indole test was negative and the lysine decarboxylase and urease tests positive. These three tests precisely differentiate the three organisms.
8. In addition to the above, the organism showed the following reactions, which further confirm its identity:
   (a) citrate utilization: positive,
   (b) oxidase production: negative,
   (c) nitrate reduction: positive.

Organism: *Enterobacter*

Sensitivity

Furaltadone, S
Neomycin, S
Penicillin, R
Streptomycin, R
Sulfathiazole, R
Terramycin, R
Tetracycline, R

Case 10

Species: Canine, adult male

History/Diagnosis: Chronic nasal discharge

Specimen: Nasal swab

Laboratory Findings

1. No growth occurred on MacConkey agar.
2. On blood agar there was a light growth of medium-sized, almost colorless, nonhemolytic colonies.
3. The Gram stain showed gram-negative coccobacilli mixed with bacilli.
4. Growth on TSI agar produced yellow butt, with no H_2S production.
5. Other tests showed oxidase production, indole production, and no urease production.
6. *Pasteurella multocida* is often definitely rod-shaped. The early observation of coccobacillic morphology could have been misleading. With the general growth characteristics and biochemical reactions, the problem was to differentiate between *Pasteurella multocida* from *Pasteurella pneumotropica.*

Organism: *Pasteurella multocida*

Sensitivity

Aureomycin, R
Chloromycetin, S
Furadantin, R
Kanamycin, S
Neomycin, S

Penicillin, S
Polymyxin B, S
Terramycin, S

Case 11

Species: Equine, adult female

History/Diagnosis: Infertility

Specimen: Swab from cervix

Laboratory Findings

1. No growth was observed on MacConkey agar.
2. On blood agar light growth of large, moist, grayish-white colonies, each surrounded by a zone of green pigment, was seen.
3. Gram-negative rods.
4. Only one swab had been submitted and it had been streaked first onto blood agar. A subculture was therefore made onto MacConkey agar because the green pigment suggested *Pseudomonas*. Growth occurred promptly with colorless colonies measuring well over 1 mm in diameter after 24 hr of incubation.
5. Growth on TSI agar produced neither change in color of butt nor H_2S production.
6. On OF medium the organism showed oxidative utilization of glucose.
7. Oxidase production occurred.
8. The heavy growth on the sensitivity plate gave a noticeable "fruity" odor and green pigmentation in the surrounding agar.
9. The case illustrates poor specimen collection technique and poor plating procedure.

Organism: *Pseudomonas*

Sensitivity

Furaltadone, S
Neomycin, S
Penicillin, R
Polymyxin B, S
Streptomycin, S
Sulfathiazole, R
Terramycin, R
Tetracycline, R

Case 12

Species: Equine, adult female

History/Diagnosis: Infertility

Specimen: Cervical swab

Laboratory Findings

1. MacConkey agar culture showed a moderate growth of large pink colonies considerably over 1 mm in diameter and appearing very mucoid.
2. Blood agar culture showed moderate growth of large "dirty white" nonhemolytic colonies.
3. On inoculated TSI, no H_2S was produced. The butt was acidified.
4. Inoculated SIM agar showed no indole production. The stab line showed no motility.
5. Lysine decarboxylase reaction was positive.
6. In addition to the above, the organism showed the following reactions:
   (a) citrate: positive,
   (b) urease: positive.

Organism: *Klebsiella* sp.

Sensitivity

Furaltadone, S
Neomycin, S
Penicillin, —
Streptomycin, S
Sulfathiazole, S
Terramycin, S
Tetracycline, S

Case 13

Species Equine, four-month-old female

History/Diagnosis: Diarrhea

Specimen: Rectal swab

Laboratory Findings

1. Two colony types were seen on the MacConkey agar plate after overnight incubation, both types exceeding 1 mm in diameter:

(a) moderate growth of pink to red colonies,
(b) heavy growth of colorless colonies.

2. Blood agar growth was not remarkable.
3. The organism arbitrarily called (a) above gave the following biochemical reactions:
   (a) TSI: no H_2S, acid butt,
   (b) indole: positive,
   (c) citrate: negative,
   (d) urease: negative.

Organism: *Escherichia*

4. The (b) organism reacted as follows:
   (a) TSI: H_2S produced,
   (b) urease: negative,
   (c) lysine decarboxylase production: positive,
   (d) malonate utilization: negative.

In addition to the results of the above tests, which are considered the minimum prior to testing with *Salmonella* 0 polyvalent antiserum, the organism showed these reactions:
   (a) indole production: negative,
   (b) citrate utilization: positive.

5. A suspension of the organism was agglutinated by *Salmonella* 0 polyvalent A-1 antiserum.

Organism: *Salmonella* sp.

Sensitivity of Salmonella

Furaltadone, S
Neomycin, —
Penicillin, —
Streptomycin, —
Sulfathiazole, —
Terramycin, —
Tetracycline, —

Case 14

Species: Equine

History/Diagnosis: Inguinal abscess

Specimen: Exudate from abscess, plated directly onto blood agar and into thioglycolate broth

Laboratory Findings

1. Direct smear showed a variety of morphological types, one of which showed marked pleomorphism.
2. After four days of anaerobic incubation, two gram-negative organisms (A and B) were recovered from blood agar culture and one from thioglycolate broth. Organism A was a pleomorphic gram-negative bacillus which showed swollen forms. Organism B was a uniform gram-negative bacillus with rounded ends. Colonies of B were distinguished from those of A by being nonhemolytic.
3. Upon repeated subcultures, A became more uniform. It always showed distinct beta hemolysis.
4. Organism B was found to have specific nutritional requirements provided by blood; liquid media did not support its growth.
5. Neither organism would grow on PEA. Although this medium contains blood, it inhibits gram-negative organisms.
6. Neither organism A nor B would grow in microaerophilic or aerobic atmospheres.
7. Both organisms produced distinctly foul odors.
8. Organism A gave the following reactions after four days of incubation: catalase production and nitrate reduction were negative; glucose, lactose, maltose, and sucrose were fermented.
9. Organism B was found to neither produce catalase nor reduce indole. Its fastidious nutritional requirements were not provided in the differential media, and its biochemical profile was not determined. The rounded ends on the bacilli indicated *Bacteroides* rather than *Fusobacterium.*

Organism A: *Sphaerophorus necrophorus*

Organism B: *Bacterioides* sp.

Sensitivity

	A	B		A	B
Aureomycin	S	S	Furaltadone	S	S
Chloromycetin	S	S	Sulfathiazole	S	R
Furadantin	S	S	Sulfamethizole	R	R
Kanamycin	R	R	Terramycin	S	S
Neomycin	R	R	Tetracycline	S	R
Penicillin	S	R	Tylosin	S	R
Polymixin B	S	R	Streptomycin	R	R

Case 15

Species: Equine, five years old

History/Diagnosis: Abscess in socket of upper right premolar tooth

Specimen: Swab for anaerobic and aerobic culture

Laboratory Findings

1. After three days of anaerobic incubation, nonhemolytic colonies were observed on blood agar.
2. Organism showed as gram-positive cocci in long chain formations.
3. No growth was obtained from initial swabs in aerobic culture.
4. The cocci were strictly anaerobic when subcultured.
5. Good colony development was obtained on blood agar and PEA in three days of incubation. No growth occurred on trypticase soy or MacConkey agar.
6. The organism did not produce catalase.
7. Other tests showed fermentation with gas production from lactose, sucrose, and maltose. Glucose was not attacked.
8. The organism reduced nitrate but did not produce indole.
9. It was nonmotile.

Organism: *Peptostreptococcus anaerobius*

Sensitivity

Aureomycin, S
Chloromycetin, S
Furadantin, S
Kanamycin, S
Neomycin, R
Penicillin, S
Polymixin B, R
Terramycin, S

Case 16

Species: Canine

History/Diagnosis: Abortion

Specimen: Swab from peritoneum of aborted fetus

Laboratory Findings

1. Direct microscopic examination showed gram-positive bacilli.
2. No aerobic growth occurred in seven days.
3. Two strict anaerobes were isolated: (A) gram-positive bacilli showing as spreading, beta hemolytic colonies which appeared dark by transmitted light; (B) gram-positive bacilli, slender and longer than (A), showing as beta hemolytic, nonspreading colonies which appeared colorless by transmitted light.
4. The organisms had the following characteristics:

Characteristic	Medium	A	B
Atmospheric requirements	air	−	−
	microaerophilic	−	−
	anaerobic	+	+
Nutritional requirements	trypticase soy agar	slight growth	slight growth
	PEA	fair growth	fair growth
	blood agar	good growth	good growth
Carbohydrate fermentation	glucose	+	+
	lactose	+	+
	sucrose	+	−
	salicin	−	+
Catalase production		−	−
Nitrate reduction		+	+
Indole production		−	−
Gelatin liquification		+	+

Organism A: *Clostridium chauvoei*

Organism B: *Clostridium septicum*

These two species of *Clostridium* are differentiated on the basis of fermentation of sucrose and salicin.

Sensitivity

	A	B		A	B
Aureomycin	S	—	Polymixin B	R	R
Chloromycetin	S	S	Furaltadone	S	S
Furadantin	S	S	Sulfathiazole	S	R
Kanamycin	R	R	Sulfamerizole	S	R
Neomycin	R	R	Terramycin	S	S
Penicillin	S	S	Tetracycline	S	S

Case 17

Species: Equine, three weeks old

History/Diagnosis: Diarrhea

Specimen: Fecal swab

Laboratory Findings

1. After overnight incubation the MacConkey plate contained a heavy growth of lactose fermenting (red) colonies all well in excess of 1 mm in diameter.
2. The blood agar plate showed: (A) a heavy growth of medium-sized nonhemolytic organisms numerically comparable with the lactose-fermenting growth on MacConkey agar; (B) moderate numbers of alpha hemolytic streptococci; (C) many medium-sized, nearly transparent, sparkling, beta hemolytic colonies.
3. When organism C was subcultured onto MacConkey agar the organism grew poorly and produced barely visible red colonies in 48 hr.
4. When organism C was subcultured for isolation onto blood agar, it showed only slight alpha hemolysis. The colonies were now dry in appearance. All subsequent subculturing failed to produce the smooth form seen on the original plate.
5. In its smooth form the organism appeared as gram-negative cocci to filamentous bacilli. Smears from rough colonies showed the bacilli to be thinner with increased pleomorphism.
6. Organism C was nonmotile and produced oxidase and urease. These reactions, together with the slow growth and lactose-fermenting colonies, indicated that the organism was *actino bacillus*. In addition to the characteristics given above, it was found to reduce nitrate and ferment glucose, but it did not utilize citrate.

Organism: *Actinobacillus equuli*

Sensitivity

Furaltadone, S
Neomycin, R
Penicillin, R
Streptomycin, R
Terramycin, R
Tetracycline, R

Case 18

Species: Ovine

History/Diagnosis: Pneumonia, caseous lymphadenitis

Specimen: Swab from prefemoral lymph node abscess

Laboratory Findings

1. After 36 hr of incubation a heavy growth of small white colonies in pure culture was observed. The colonies showed incomplete beta hemolysis.
2. No growth was observed on MacConkey agar.
3. Microscopic appearance of Gram-stained preparation from blood agar showed gram-positive cocci; but when the organism was grown in trypticase soy broth for sensitivity testing, the stained preparation showed thin medium-length rods.
4. The organism produced catalase.
5. It was studied intensively and confirmed to be *Corynebacterium ovis*.

Organism: *Corynebacterium ovis*

Sensitivity

Furaltadone, R
Neomycin, R
Penicillin, S
Sulfamerazole, R
Terramycin, S
Tetracycline, S

Index

M

N

T